ANATOMY OF CRUDE DRUGS

12th edition

Prof. Dr. M. A. IYENGAR

and

S. G. K. NAYAK

Former Faculty

Department of Pharmacognosy

Manipal College of Pharmaceutical Sciences

MANIPAL – 576 104

INDIA

PharmaMed Press

An imprint of BSP Books Pvt. Ltd.

4-4-309/316, Giriraj Lane,

Sultan Bazar, Hyderabad - 500 095

ANATOMY OF CRUDE DRUGS

ISBN: 978-81-7800-290-3 (Paperback)

Published by

PharmaMed Press

An imprint of BSP Books Pvt. Ltd.

4-4-309/316, Giriraj Lane, Sultan Bazar, Hyderabad - 500 095

Phone: 23445688; Fax: 91+40-23445611

E-mail: info@pharmamedpress.com

www.bspbooks.net/pharmamedpress.net

Price: Rs. 100/-

First Edition	:	1975
Second Edition	:	1979
Third Edition	:	1984
Fourth Edition	:	1987
Fifth Edition	:	1991
Sixth Edition	:	1994
Seventh Edition	:	1998
Eighth Edition	:	2001
Ninth Edition	:	2004
Tenth Edition	:	2006
Eleventh Edition	:	2008
Twelfth Edition	:	2011

2025 *Thirteenth Reprint*

PREFACE TO THIRTEENTH EDITION:

The continued survival in the hands of pharmacy students at large, in spite of the stealthy competition, speaks of its popularity, originality and quality. Thanks to all concerned.

AUTHORS

CONTENTS

FUNDAMENTALS OF PLANT ANATOMY

(No exhaustive coverage of the fundamental aspects of Plant Anatomy is attempted here. Nevertheless, care has been taken to provide essential and relevant explanations confined only to the drugs included here.)

Robert Hooke, the English Microscopist coined the word CELL in the 17th century to the fundamental unit of a plant body or an organic structure. The word cell is derived from Latin where 'Cellula' means a small compartment. Katherine Esau, one of the leading Plant Anatomist of our times defines in her worthy book 'Plant Anatomy' the cell as "a protoplast with or without a non-living envelope, the cell wall, and consisting of the protoplasmic components and non-protoplasmic materials, the latter intimately connected with the vital activities of the protoplast."

Group of cells with same form and function is called a TISSUE. The cell membrane of two neighbouring cells in a tissue is connected through a pectin layer called middle lamella. The cell wall, cell membrane, protoplasm and as well the middle lamella give out fine protoplasmic threads called PLASMODESMATA. These cytoplasmic threads interconnect the protoplasm of different cells and thus help in conduction and communication of food and stimuli respectively.

Groups of tissues showing common features and some continuity are called TISSUE SYSTEMS.

Tissue Systems are classified as follows:

1. Dermal (Outer protective covering like epidermis, periderm, etc.)
2. Fundamental (ground tissue made of collenchyma, parenchyma, etc.)
3. Vascular (stelar structures like phloem and xylem).

Dermal Tissue System: EPIDERMIS is the outermost protective, uniseriate layer of the young plant body. The epidermal cells are closely placed and show wide variation in size, shape and arrangement with no intercellular spaces. Epidermal cells are often covered on the outer side with a thin or thick layer of cuticle which is impervious and contains chemical substance called 'cutin'. Roots do not possess cuticle for obvious reasons.

Dermal or Epidermal Tissue System includes (particularly in leaves):

a) **Stomata** (pores or openings) and b) **Trichomes** (hairs). **Stomata** (sing-stoma): A stoma is made of a pair of identical cells called guard cells placed parallel to each other and also form a pore in the centre through which gaseous exchange takes place. The epidermal cells surrounding the stoma are called subsidiary cells and look at times different from the other epidermal cells. Four different types of stomata occur based on their arrangement with the subsidiary cells. RANUNCULACEOUS or ANOMOCYTIC (irregular celled) type of stoma meaning thereby that the subsidiary cells surrounding the stomal pore are irregularly arranged and cannot be differentiated from other epidermal cells. CRUCIFEROUS or ANISOCYTIC (unequal celled) type of stoma meaning thereby that the stomal pore is surrounded by 3 epidermal cells (subsidiary cells) of which one is invariably smaller than the other two. RUBIACEOUS or PARACYTIC (parallel celled) type meaning thereby that the two subsidiary cells are parallel to that of stoma. CARYOPHYLLACEOUS or DIACYTIC (cross celled) type of stoma meaning thereby the two subsidiary cells are at right angles to that of stoma.

These different types of stomata are very specific and thus act as diagnostic characters.

Trichomes: These are epidermal appendages. A trichome can normally be differentiated into a base embedded in the epidermal cell and a tube like projecting body. Normally the trichomes are of two types. a) Covering and b) Glandular. Both covering and glandular trichomes may be unicellular or multicellular, uniseriate or multiseriate and stalked or sessile. Covering trichomes have protective function, whereas glandular trichomes have taken up the function of secretion of essential oils or oleo-resins.

PERIDERM: The epidermis in mature plant parts (stem and root) gets substituted by periderm which results due to the activity of the meristematic tissue called *Phellogen* or *Cork cambium*. Certain cells below the epidermis in a young plant take up new form and function as a result of stelar secondary growth. This newly formed 1 or 2 layers of phellogen divides and redivides to form *Phellem* or *Cork* on the outer side and *Phelloderm* on the inner side. The cork cells are seen in a t.s. as rectangular or brick shaped, compact, the walls being impregnated with a substance called 'suberin'. Phelloderm cells are mostly parenchymatous in nature. Phellem, phellogen and phelloderm are collectively called as periderm. LENTICELS are pores identical in function to stomata but occur in periderm. The only difference between stomal pore and lenticel is that stomal pore is regulated by the living guard cells on either side and as a result the pore may be large or small in its dimension whereas the lenticel, in the absence of the guard cells, remains permanently open.

Fundamental or Ground Tissue System: This is restricted usually to hypodermis, cortex, pith and in case of leaves mesophyll and a portion of midrib and comprises of the following tissues.

PARENCHYMA contains cells which are living, thin walled with intercellular spaces. The shape often varies and these are found in the cortex of root, cortex and pith of stem and mesophyll of leaf. Some parenchyma may also show pitted and reticulate thickenings which however are exception to the rule. Chlorenchyma is Parenchyma containing chloroplasts. Aerenchyma is Parenchyma with large intercellular spaces.
Function: Storage, photosynthesis etc.

COLLENCHYMA contains cells which are also living. The cells resemble parenchyma but the cell walls at the corners get thickened with cellulose. This tissue occurs mostly in the cortical region of stem, petiole, bark and midrib of a leaf.
Function: Mechanical strength.

SCLERENCHYMA is a dead tissue. The cell walls are heavily thickened with "lignin", hence it is also called a lignified tissue. They occur in all parts of the plant body where mechanical strength is needed.

Further, this sclerenchyma may occur either in the form of fibres which are elongate sclerenchyma cells or in the form of short isodiametric or irregular cells called stone-cells or sclereids.

Stone cells may occur either singly or in bands. They are heavily lignified with varying lumen (the middle space left over after the lignification). They also vary in shape and size. They provide valuable diagnostic characters.

Sclerenchymatous fibres are narrow, often elongated (as much as 20 cms) with pointed ends. The cell walls are usually lignified. These also help in the identification of crude drugs and as well given mechanical support to plants.

VASCULAR TISSUE SYSTEM: This complex tissue is responsible for the conduction of food material and water. Phloem a living tissue conducts food material from leaves to the different parts of the plant body whereas xylem a dead tissue conducts water from roots to leaves.

PHLOEM normally consists of phloem parenchyma, sieve tubes and companion cells. Phloem fibres also occur in some plants.

XYLEM usually consists of xylem (wood) parenchyma, trachea (vessels), tracheids and xylem (wood) fibres. Xylem parenchyma helps in storage, wood fibres in mechanical support and trachea and tracheids in actual conduction of water.

TRACHEIDS are elongated tubes pointed at both ends and frequently cut across with oblique walls with perforations.

TRACHEA are also elongated tubes like tracheids but without any oblique perforated walls.

The earlier formed xylem is called as PROTOXYLEM and the later formed METAXYLEM (not to be confused with primary and secondary xylem). Based on the position of protoxylem, a t.s. of stem or root can be distinguished. In case of stem, groups of protoxylem point to the centre, a condition called 'endarch' whereas in a root, protoxylem groups point towards the periphery leading to an 'exarch' condition. Further, based on the number of protoxylem groups, terms like 'monarch', 'diarch', 'triarch', 'pentarch' and 'polyarch' are used. In dicot roots the protoxylem bundles vary from 2 to 6 or in other words diarch to hexarch whereas in monocot roots the number of protoxylem groups are more than 10 and as a result a polyarch condition is reached.

Annular, spiral, reticulate, scalariform and pitted are the various types of thickenings of the tracheary elements. These thickenings, to a certain extent help as diagnostic characters as they are specific in their distribution.

Xylem and Phloem are associated to form a VASCULAR BUNDLE.

According to the mode of occurrence of xylem and phloem, the vascular bundles are of the following types:

1. **Collateral:** This is the most common type of vascular bundle in the stems and leaves. Here xylem and phloem remain side by side arranged on the same radius, phloem on the outerside and xylem on the inner side. Collateral bundles may be open (cambium present in between phloem and xylem) or closed (cambium absent).
2. **Bicollateral:** These are collateral bundles, but have in addition to external phloem, another patch of phloem on the inner side which may be called internal phloem.
3. **Concentric:** Here one kind of vascular tissue surrounds the other.
4. **Radial:** These bundles are fundamentally different from the types mentioned above, in view of the fact that here xylem and phloem occur in separate patches, on alternate radii on the axix. Radial vascular bundles are characteristic of roots.

In dicot stems the vascular bundles are arranged in the form of a ring and in monocot, the bundles are scattered. Thus by looking at the arrangement of the bundles, a dicot or monocot stem can be distinguished. In leaves, vascular bundles are seen in transverse view only in the midrib. Depending on the type of venation, vascular strands are cut either obliquely and in various planes (dicot plants with reticulate venation) or transversely (as in monocots with parallel venation).

CAMBIUM is a meristematic tissue present between the phloem and xylem in dicot stems. In young roots the cambium is absent but as the plant matures a strip of cambium appears between the radially placed phloem and xylem which ultimately forms a zig-zag ring giving out secondary xylem on the inner-side and secondary phloem on the outer side. In stems the interfascicular and the intrafascicular join together also to form a ring and divide and re-divide to yield secondary phloem to the exterior and secondary xylem towards the interior. Because of the appearance of these secondary structures, the delicate primary structures are either crushed and disintegrated or poorly represented in mature plant parts. The components of secondary phloem and secondary xylem are very similar to primary structures.

MEDULLARY RAYS consisting of parenchymatous cells run diagonally and extend from pith (medulla) to the cortex through the secondary xylem and secondary phloem. Width of the rays may vary from 1 (uni-) to many (multiseriate). These rays are very well seen in all the barks and as well in wood.

Function: Conduction of food material and water in the lateral directions.

Excretory Products: Calcium oxalate crystals found in plant parts which occur in 5 different forms are considered as excretory products. These provide valuable information in the identification of drugs. Prisms of calcium oxalate may occur singly or in small groups. Cluster crystals also called as Sphaeraphides, Druses are spherical aggregates of sharp pointed angular crystals. Acicular Raphides are needle shaped occurring singly but often in bundles enclosed in a bundle sheath. Microsphenoidal crystals or also called fine sandy crystals occur like an amorphous mass in a cell.

Cystoliths are aggregates of crystals made of calcium carbonate. These appear as small bunches of grapes whose stalks are made of cellulose.

Secretory Products: Essential oils, oleo-resin, latex etc., are secretory products and are present, in special tissues like oil-cell layer, glandular trichome, laticiferous ducts, etc.

Three types of secretory cavities are known: Schizogenous (cavities formed because of the splitting of the epithelial cells which can be easily made out by the regularity of the cavity). Lysigenous, where the cavity formed is due to the dissolution of cells (hence an irregular cavity is formed) and Schizolysigenous cavity is formed because of the operation of both mentioned above.

Methodical Approach: While examining the microscopic sections of ROOT and RHIZOME DRUGS the following important points are to be observed.

1. The arrangement of vascular bundles and the type of the vascular bundle.
2. Size, type and thickenings of vessels and fibres.
3. Width and nature of medullary ray cells.
4. Presence or absence of stone cells; if present then the type, shape and size.

5. Type of cork cells.
6. Endodermal layer (*endodermis* is the innermost cortical layer) and nature of its cells.
7. Type and size of starch grains when present.
8. Type and form of calcium oxalate crystals.
9. If possible, locate the tissues containing the active principles.

BARK DRUGS

1. Details of periderm which includes phellem, phellogen and phelloderm.
2. Cortex and its cellular contents.
3. Bast (phloem) fibres, if any.
4. Size and shape of stone cells (sclereids) when present.
5. Type of calcium oxalate crystals when present.
6. Cells containing essential oil etc.
7. Width of medullary rays.
8. If possible, location of the active principles.

WOOD DRUGS

1. Type of vessels and various thickenings.
2. Height and width of medullary rays cells.
3. Type of fibres.
4. Type of crystals, if any.
5. If possible location of the active principles or the elements containing them.

LEAF DRUGS

1. Whether a leaf is dorsiventral or isobilateral.
2. If trichomes are present then their types and form.
3. Type of stomata.
4. Epidermal layer with its cells.
5. Arrangement of palisade and spongy parenchyma.
6. Details of the midrib.
7. Excretory and Secretory products, if any.
8. Location of active principles or the tissues containing them, when possible.

Surface preparations are taken in case of leaves to study the epidermal cells in surface view, trichomes and stomata.

FLOWER DRUGS: Normally no t.s. is taken to study a flower drug. All the same, a vertical section is taken to study the different parts of a flower. Clove being a flower bud, a t.s. of interest and the details appear under clove elsewhere.

FRUIT and SEED DRUGS: The outer covering of the fruit which is called as PERICARP is distinguished into outer epicarp, middle mesocarp and inner endocarp. The outermost layer of seed is the testa which encloses the endosperm (at times perisperm) which in turn encloses the embryo. The endosperm and perisperm are nutritive tissues. Endosperm is formed inside the embryo sac whereas perisperm is formed outside the embryo sac, that is, in other words is derived from nucellus. Shape and cellular contents of endosperm and type of endosperm and embryo cells are of importance, besides the epidermal layer of testa and other neighbouring layers.

MOUNTING: Thinnnest possible section of a plant part is taken on a slide and mounted in a solution of chloral hydrate. On slightly warming, the section gets cleared in the presence of chloral hydrate. Cover the section carefully with a cover glass taking care no air bubbles creep in. Glycerin could also be used as a mounting medium and the sections in glycerin remain fresh for a long time.

STAINING: In order to differentiate the tissues, the sections are to be stained. This is done by treating section for 1 or 2 minutes with 1:1 mixture of phloroglucinol and con. Hydrochloric acid. Lignified tissues, like xylem, sclerenchyma, etc., because of the lignifications take up red colour.

TEST FOR STARCH: Mount a section on a slide in WATER. Irrigate the section with dil. Iodine. Starch turns blue with iodine.

TEST FOR FIXED OIL: Mount a section containing fixed oil in Sudan III. On warming, fixed oil acquires an orange yellow colour.

TEST FOR MUCILAGE: Mucilage present in various tissues, turns pink with Ruthenium Red Solution.

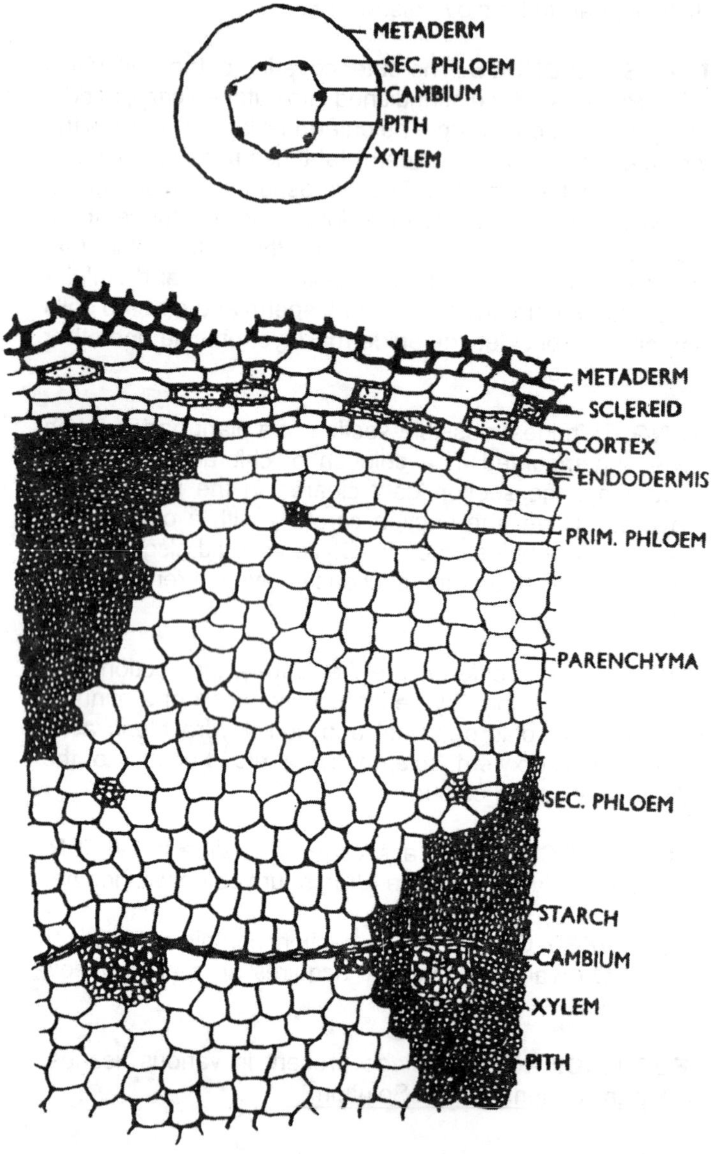

Aconite Root. Diagrammatic and an enlarged portion of T. S. (X 100)

TUBERA ACONITI (*Aconitum napellus* L.)

T.S. of a tuberous root presents a circular outline with a wavy margin. The following tissues are observed from the periphery to the centre.

METADERM the epidermis or the epiblema is usually not seen. However, few layers of cortical cells become suberized and take up the protective function. Hence this tissue gets the term – mataderm – and its cells are tangentially elongated, thick walled and brownish in colour.

PRIMARY CORTEX 4 to 6 layered with tangentially elongated, thin walled parenchymatous cells. Interspersed with this tissue are the stone cells which are often isolated, sometimes in groups, rectangular to subrectangular, thick walled, lignified and pitted with large lumen.

ENDODERMIS distinct, single layered with tangentially elongated parenchymatous cells having suberized walls.

PHLOEM occupies relatively a large area, with thick walled, big parenchymatous cells which are densely packed with starch. Groups of sieve elements representing the primary phloem are seen scattered in the parenchyma below endodermis. Groups of sieve tissues of secondary phloem are found in the parenchyma just above the cambium ring, usually opposite to the xylem groups.

CAMBIUM 2 – 3 layered, more or less in the form of a stellate ring.

XYLEM is represented in several discontinuous groups of vessels immediately below the angles of cambium. The vessels show largely reticulate and pitted thickenings although spiral and annular thickenings are not uncommon.

PITH large, parenchymatous, cells are radially elongated to isodiametric and contain abundant starch.

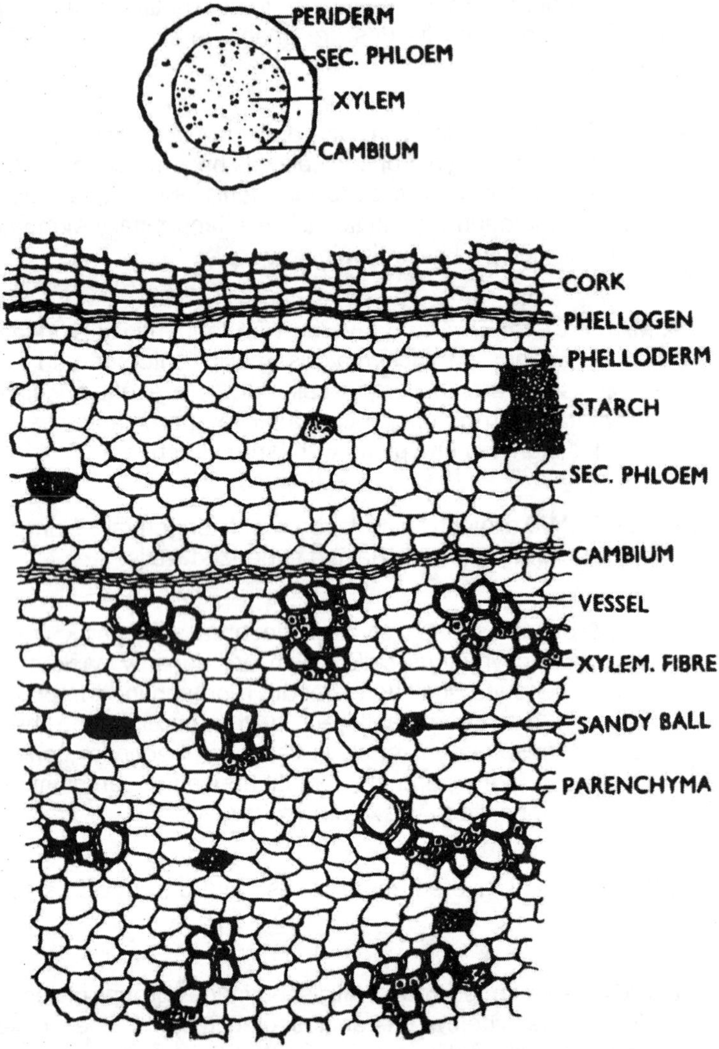

Belladonna Root. Diagrammatic and an enlarged portion of T. S. (X 100)

RADIX BELLADONNAE

(*Atropa acuminata* Royle ex Lindley)

T.S. of a somewhat young root which is circular in outline with wavy margin, shows broadly from the periphery to the centre, periderm, secondary phloem, cambium and a bulky porous secondary xylem.

PERIDERM is distinguishable into phellem (cork) and phelloderm.

Cork few layers, cells tangentially elongated and arranged in radial rows.

Phellogen not distinguishable though a faint layer can be made out.

Phelloderm few layers, cells tangentially elongated and contain starch and yellowish matter. Besides a few groups of the crystalline sand of calcium oxalate (sandy balls) are seen occasionally in the phelloderm region.

SECONDARY PHLOEM several layers of starch bearing parenchyma with groups of sieve elements. Phloem fibres absent. Numerous sandy balls, a characteristic feature of Belladonna root and leaf, are seen scattered throughout in the phloem tissue.

CAMBIUM is represented in the form of a ring containing 4 to 5 layers of rectangular cells arranged in radial rows.

SECONDARY XYLEM forms the bulk of the root and occupies a large area. Secondary xylem consists of largely starch bearing parenchyma with several scattered groups of vessels (3 to 10), associated with tracheids, fibres and cellulosic parenchyma. The goups of vessels are more towards the cambium. Primary xylem forming the central mass shows distinct diarch nature. As in phloem, here too numerous characteristic sandy balls are seen all over the xylem parenchyma.

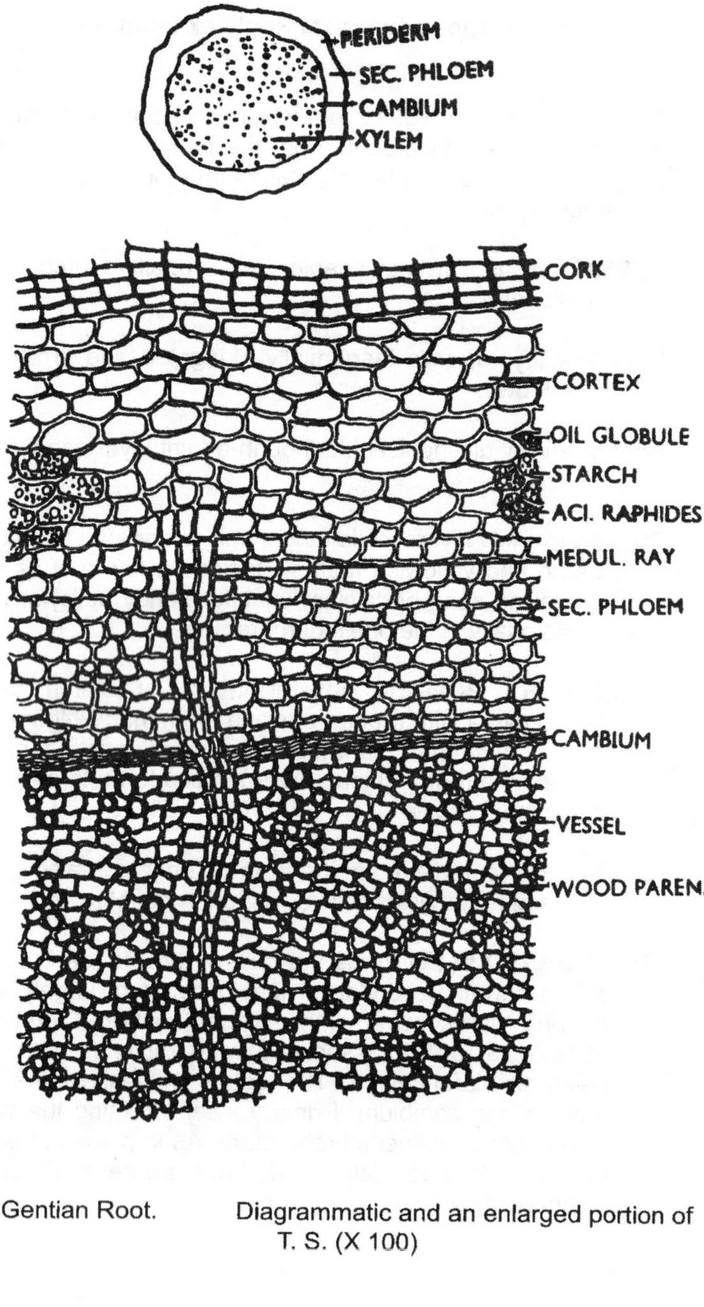

Gentian Root. Diagrammatic and an enlarged portion of T. S. (X 100)

RADIX GENTIAN (*Gentiana lutea* L.)

A t.s. of the root is more or less circular with wavy margin. The following tissues are seen from the periphery to the centre.

PERIDERM

Cork 4 to 6 layers, thin walled rectangular cells and orange brown in colour.

Phellogen and Phelloderm not distinguishable though a few layers of thick walled tangentially elongated parenchyma is seen immediately below cork.

CORTEX thin zone of tangentially elongated thick walled parenchymatous cells containing oil globules, few starch grains and minute acicular raphides.

SECONDARY PHLOEM relatively a wider zone, made of tangentially elongated thick walled parenchymatous cells containing oil globules, few starch grains and minute acicular raphides, sieve elements are indistinct and phloem fibres are entirely absent.

CAMBIUM distinct and represented by a yellow ring of 3 to 5 layers of thin walled, small rectangular cells.

SECONDARY XYLEM forms the bulk of the root. Consists of largely parenchyma, vessels and medullary rays. The vessels are occasionally isolated but mostly in groups. Groups of vessels appear more towards the cambium. Wavy, yellowish bands of medullary rays, though indistinct, traverse the xylem parenchyma and at times extend upto the cortex. Wood fibres absent. Xylem parenchyma and medullary ray cells also contain oil globules, few starch grains and minute acicular raphides.

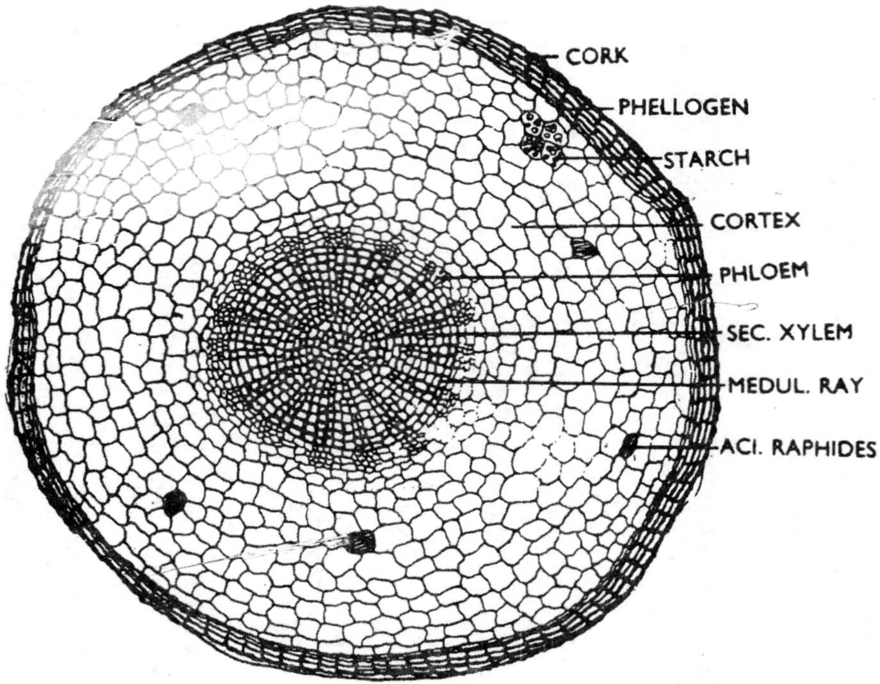

Ipecac Root. T. S. (X 100)

RADIX IPECAC

[*Cephaelis ipecacuanha* (Brot.) A. Rich]

T.S. of root shows a circular outline and the following tissues.

PERIDERM

Cork 3 to 5 layered, tangentially elongated cells filled with brown matter.

Phellogen 2 layered, immediately below the cork, shining and cells tangentially elongated.

CORTEX several layered with thin walled polyhedral parenchyma with small intercellular spaces. The cortical parenchyma contains acicular raphides either in bundles or scattered all over.

Almost every cell of the cortical parenchyma is heavily loaded with starch grains which are both simple and compound though the percentage of latter is more. Some parenchymatous cells are opalescent, which is also a characteristic feature of Valerian.

PHLOEM seen in several thin patches around the well-developed xylem and consists of perforated sieve tubes.

XYLEM occupies more or less 1/3 of the t.s. and is traversed regularly by rows of medullary rays whose cells are lignified. Because of their lignification, it is difficult to differentiate medullary rays from other wood elements in a cross section. Each ray cell, is radially elongated and contains starch. The dense secondary xylem consists of tracheids, tracheidal vessels, fibres and parenchyma. Starch grains are also seen in the xylem parenchyma.

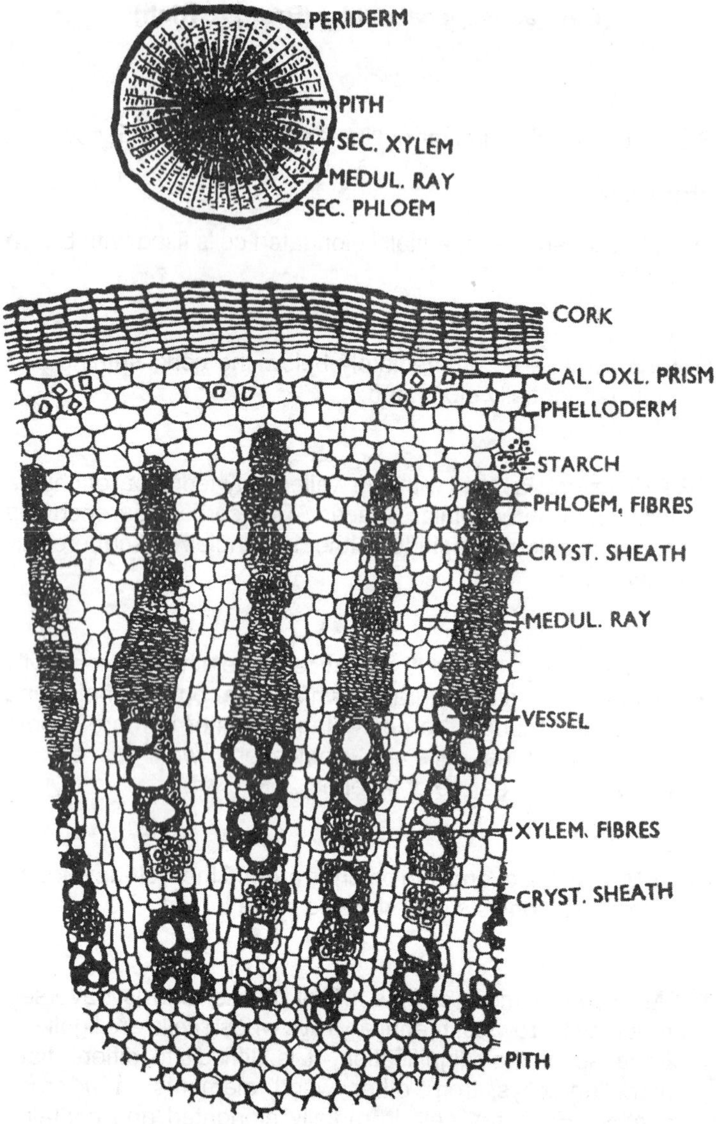

Liquorice Root (Stolon). Diagrammatic and an enlarged portion of T. S. (X 100)

RADIX LICORICE

(*Glycyrrhiza glabra* L.) (Root and Stolon)

T.S. of the stolon shows secondary features. The outline of a t.s. is more or less rounded and shows the following tissues.

PERIDERM

Phellem (cork) several layered with tabular cells; outer layers are filled with reddish brown contents and inner few are colourless.

Phellogen Indistinct.

Phelloderm 3 to 5 layered, immediately below cork, parenchymatous cells whose corners are thickened with cellulose (collenchymatous); some cells contain prisms of calcium oxalate and minute starch grains.

SECONDARY PHLOEM wide zone with numerous concentrically arranged bundles of phloem fibres. Each bundle is surrounded by a parenchymatous sheath whose cells contain prisms of calcium oxalate. Radially the fibre bundles alternate with soft phloem elements and tangentially with medullary rays.

MEDULLARY RAYS distinct, bi-to multiseriate, parenchymatous, in continuation with those of xylem. However, the rays are narrower in the xylem region and become more wider in the phloem region.

SECONDARY XYLEM well represented, divided (like phloem) by large medullary rays at regular intervals. Xylem consists of vessels, fibres and lignified wood parenchyma. The vessels which are relatively wide show scalariform the bordered pitted thickenings. Wood fibres are also ensheathed by a layer of parenchyma containing crystals. Starch is present in the wood parenchyma.

PITH consists of large parenchyma with intercellular spaces and contain few starch grains. Pith is absent in root.

Note: Root presents a very similar pattern and structural details except for pith.

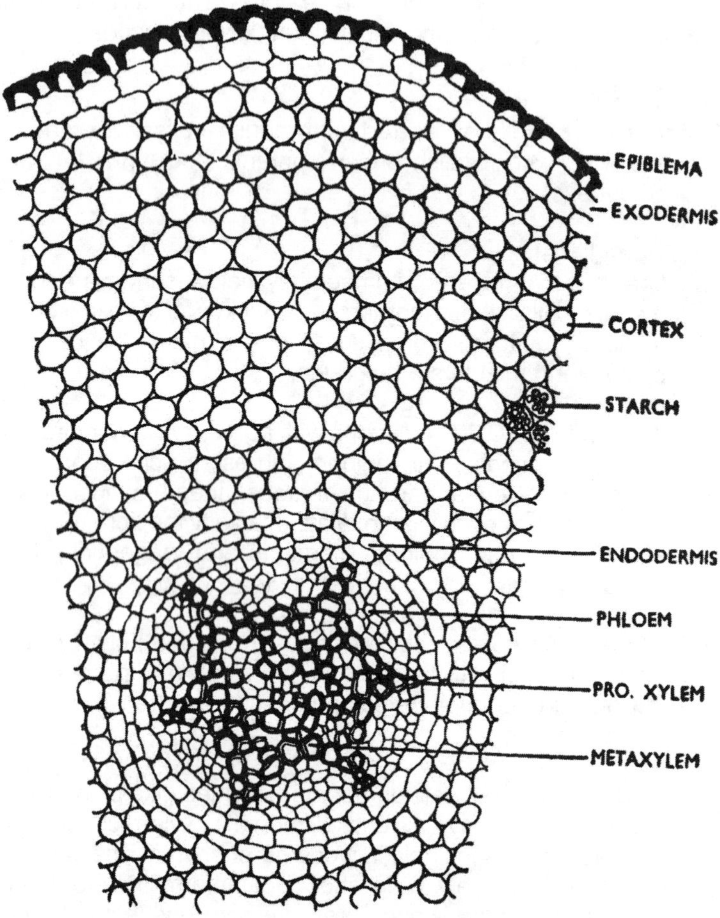

Podophyllum Root. Diagrammatic and an enlarged portion of T. S. (X 100)

RADIX PODOPHYLLI

(*Podophyllum emodi* Wall.)

The T.S. of root is circular in outline and presents the typical primary dicot root structures. The following are the tissues seen from the periphery to the centre.

EPIBLEMA single layered, yellowish brown, cells of which are slightly projecting outwards. Outer and radial walls thickened with suberin.

EXODERMIS single layered immediately below epiblema and with thin walled smaller cells.

CORTEX 18 to 22 layers of typical parenchymatous cells with wavy and pitted thick walls having intercellular spaces. They are fully loaded with starch grains but without any calcium oxalate crystals.

ENDODERMIS single layered and forms the innermost layer of cortical region. Cells are elongated with very prominent casparian strips.

VASCULAR BUNDLES
Radial, alternate, groups vary from 4 to 9 and with exarch protoxylem.

Note: When the section is taken near the rhizome, a group of sclereids are seen in the central region of the root.

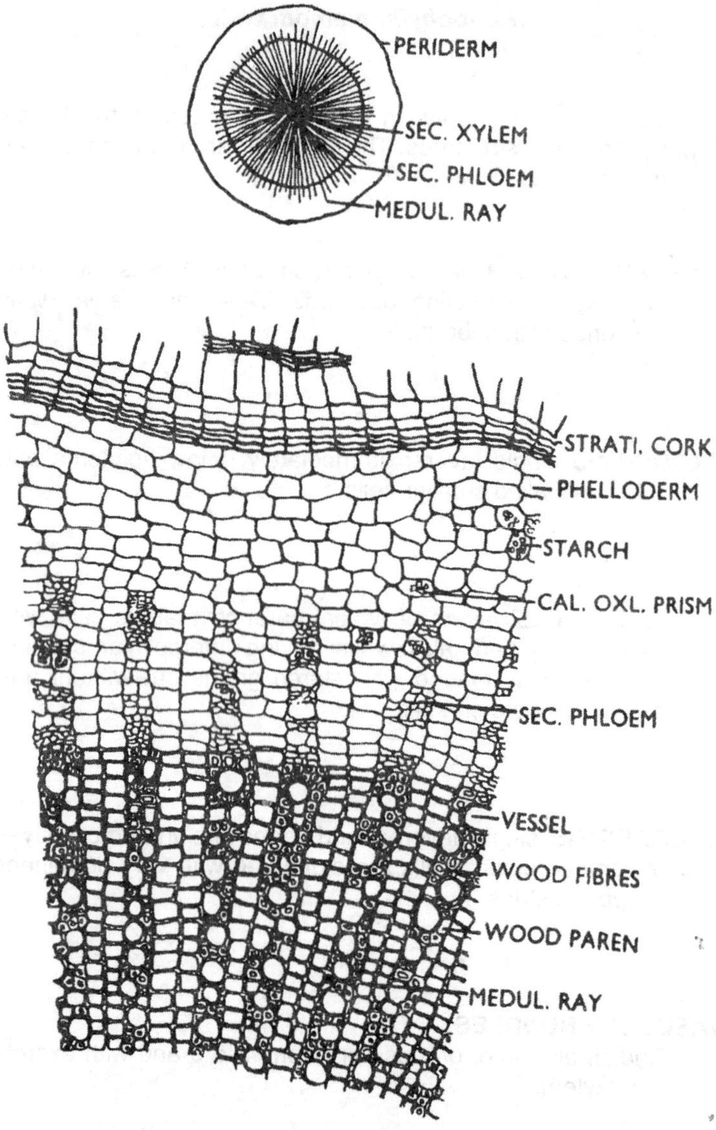

Rauwolfia Root. Diagrammatic and an enlarged portion of T. S. (X 100)

RADIX RAUWOLFIA

(*Rauwolfia serpentine* Bentham)

T.S. of the root presents a circular outline with typical stratified cork and other secondary features. Following are the tissues seen from the periphery to the centre.

PERIDERM

Cork stratified consists of alternating bands

- of smaller, suberized and un-lignified cells upto 8-10 rows in radial depth and
- of larger, suberized but lignified cells upto 5-7 rows in radial depth.

Phellogen indistinct but is seen as a narrow layer of thin walled cells.

Phelloderm 5-7 layers, immediately below the phellem, cells are arranged in radial rows whereas away from phellem, cells are oval and have intercellular spaces. Phelloderm contains abundant starch grains (with triradiate hilum) and typical twin prisms of calcium oxalate.

SECONDARY PHLOEM is traversed by conspicuous medullary rays. Phloem consists of sieve tubes, companion cells and phloem parenchyma. Starch grains and calcium oxalate prisms (as twins and groups) occur throughout the phloem tissue.

SECONDARY XYLEM is also traversed by well developed medullary rays. Xylem consists of vessels, wood fibres and lignified parenchyma. The vessels appear rounded polygonal or at times radially elongated and occur either single or in pairs. Xylem fibres appear as rounded or polygonal structures with thick lignified walls. Typical oxalate prisms and starch grains resembling those of the phelloderm and phloem occur freely in the wood parenchyma.

MEDULLARY RAYS run radially from the centre to the cortex through the phloem. Rays in the xylem region are lignified, pitted and are 1-5 cells wide although uniseriate rays are prominent. In the phloem region the ray cells are not lignified. Starch and typical oxalate prisms are present in the medullary ray cells.

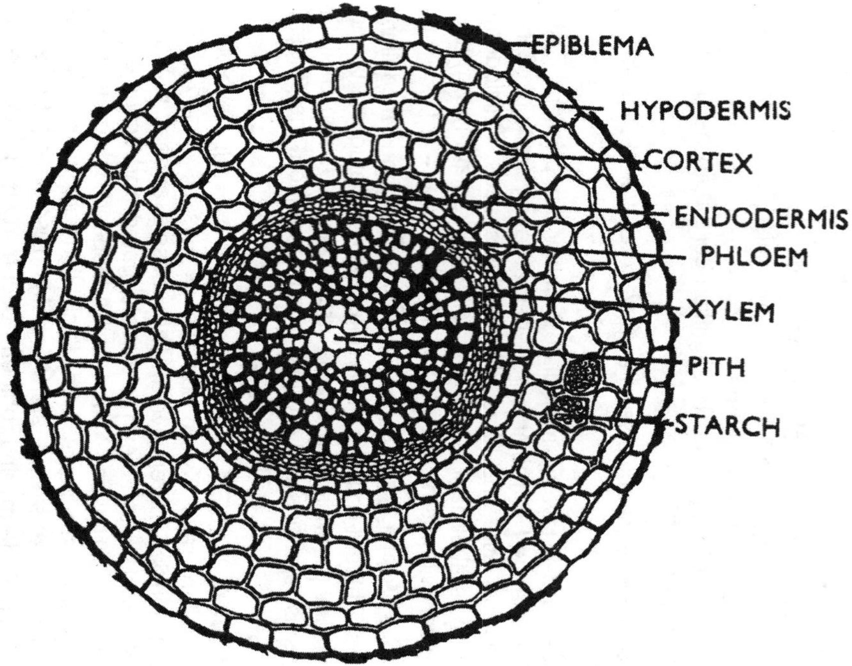

Valerian Root. T. S. (X 100)

RADIX VALERIAN

(*Valeriana Wallichii* DC.)

A t.s. of the root presents a circular outline. The following are the important tissues seen from the periphery to the centre.

EPIBLEMA outermost, indistinct, dark brown layer.

HYPODERMIS single layered, at times two layered, distinct, made of big parenchymatous cells. It is this layer which contains essential oil.

CORTEX relatively large, thick walled parenchyma containing abundant starch.

Micro reaction: With con. HCl: acetic acid 2:8 entire cortex turns blue (only in fresh sample).

ENDODERMIS innermost cortical layer, single layered, the radial walls of the cells are thickened.

VASCULAR ELEMENTS secondary features are seen only in the stelar region.

Phloem secondary phloem encircles the secondary xylem.

Xylem well developed secondary xylem with distinct vessels and lignified xylem parenchyma.

PITH small with thin walled parenchyma.

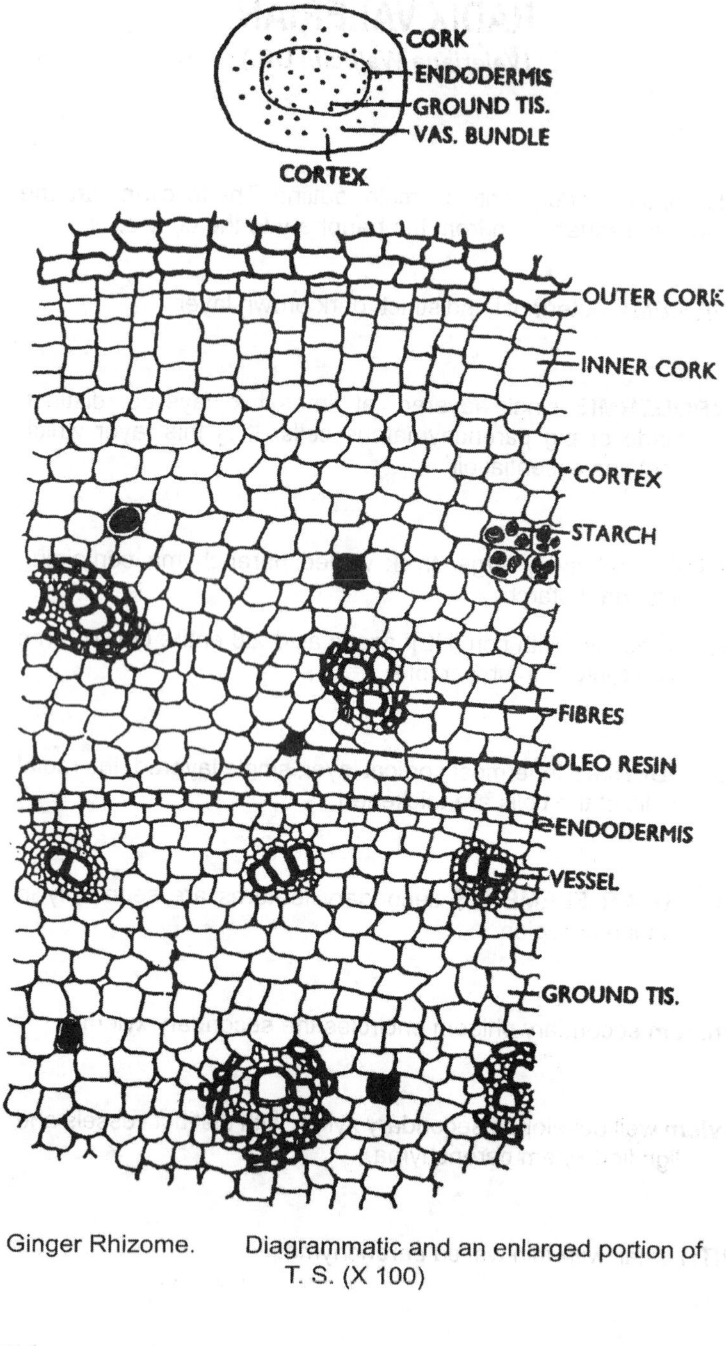

Ginger Rhizome. Diagrammatic and an enlarged portion of T. S. (X 100)

RHIZOMA ZINGIBERIS

(*Zingiber officinale* Rosoe)

A cross-section of an unpeeled mature rhizome broadly consists of the following tissues from the periphery to the centre.

CORK

Outer cork few layered, dark brown in colour, made of irregular parenchymatous cells.

Innder cork few layered, colourless parenchymatous cells radially arranged in regular rows.

CORTEX thin parenchymatous cells with intercellular spaces containing abundant starch. The starch grains are unique in the sense that they are sack shaped with terminal beak like projection in which the eccentric hilum is situated. Distinct striations are very prominent on the grain. Interspersed with cortical parenchyma are found numerous oleo-resin cells and as well vascular bundles. The oleo-resin cells have suberized walls and contain yellowish matter.

ENDODERMIS single layered with radial walls thickened and with no starch grains.

GROUND TISSUE large, parenchymatous (similar to that of cortex), with abundant starch, oleo-resin cells and vascular bundles. The latter in general are collateral, conjoint and closed. A group of sclerenchymatous fibres partially covers the vascular bundles of cortex and also of central ground tissue and these bundles are therefore called as Fibrovascular bundles. Just below the endodermal layer, that is, to the periphery of the ground tissue, a ring of narrow zone of vascular bundles appear, which however are not covered by sclerenchymatous fibres.

While the *Phloem* presents the usual well developed sieve elements, *xylem elements* are somewhat characteristic. Xylem consists of mainly vessels, some tracheids which have annular, spiral or reticulate thickenings but without any reaction for lignin. The fibres are also unlignified, pitted and septate.

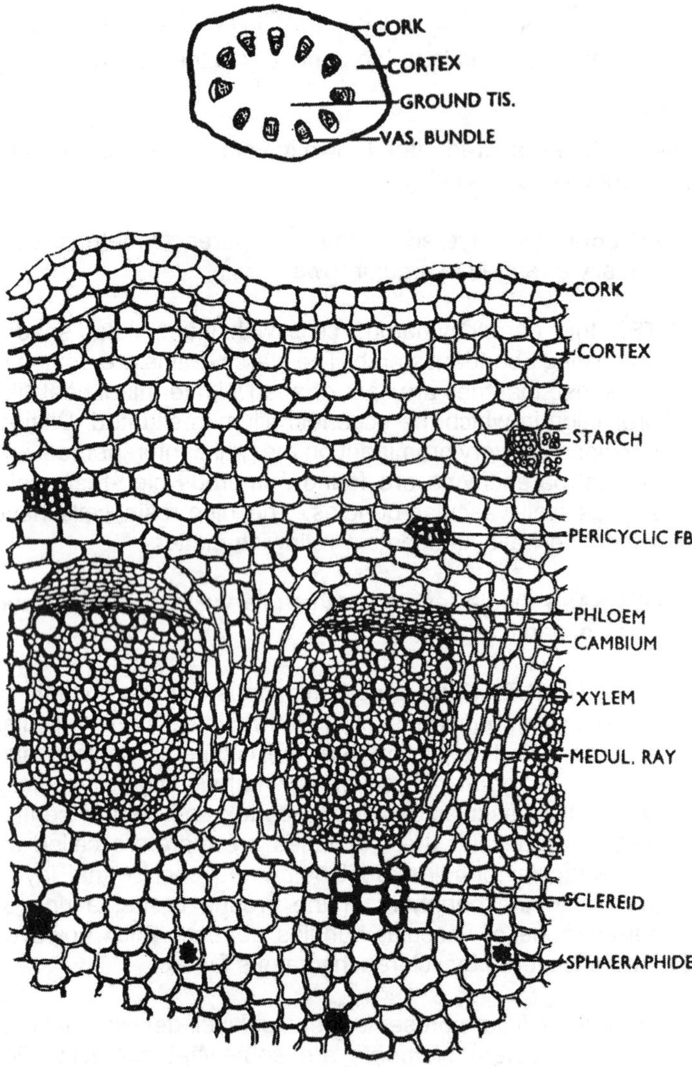

Podophyllum Rhizome. Diagrammatic and an enlarged portion of T. S. (X 100)

RHIZOMA PODOPHYLLI

(*Podophyllum emodi* Wall.)

A t.S. has an irregular outline and presents the following tissues from the periphery to the centre.

CORK 4-6 layers, polygonal cells, thin walled and contain brownish matter.

CORTEX relatively a narrow cortex, outermost 3-4 layers are of collenchymatous cells and rest parenchymatous. Cortical cells are thick walled, pitted and contain abundant starch grains.

VASCULAR BUNDLES arranged in the form of a ring, collateral, conjoint and open. Occasionally a few pericyclic fibres are seen above the phloem tissue. Phloem prominent, cambium indistinct and a well developed secondary xylem with reticulate, spiral and pitted thickenings.

Wide prominent medullarry rays are seen between the vascular bundles. Ray cells are parenchymatous, pitted, thick walled and run radially.

GROUND TISSUE large, parenchymatous and cells resemble those of cortex. Occasionally a few cells contain cluster crystals (sphaeraphides) and brown masses of resin.

Towards the peripheral region of ground tissue immediately below the vascular bundles, are seen at times some groups of pitted and thick walled stone cells.

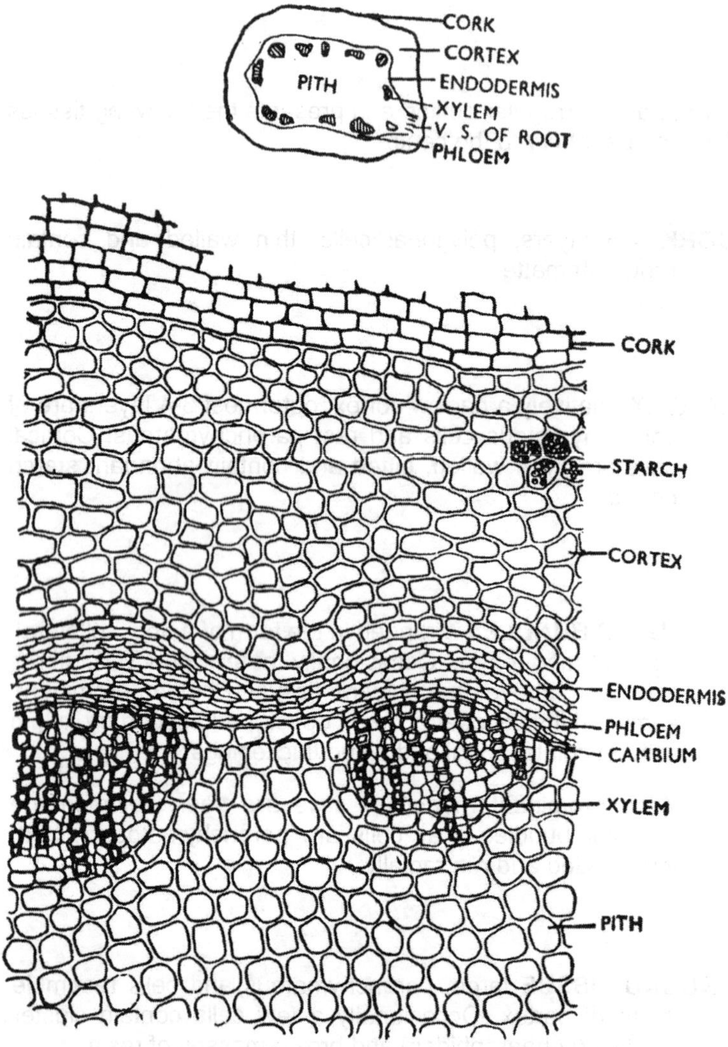

Valerian Rhizome. Diagrammatic and an enlarged portion of T. S. (X 100)

RHIZOMA VALERIAN

(*Valeriana Wallichii* DC.)

A t.s. of the rhizome presents an irregular outline and has the following tissues from periphery to centre.

CORK several layered, lignified, thin-walled with rectangular cells.

CORTEX Occupies about 1/3 of the diameter and the thick walled parenchymatous cells are fully loaded with simple starch grains. Calcium oxalate crystals are absent.

Chemical Test: Micro reaction : With con. HCl: acetic acid 2:8 entire cortex turns blue.

ENDODERMIS prominent and single layered.

VASCULAR BUNDLES 12-18, arranged in a ring, conjoint, collateral and open, phloem prominent, cambium distinct and xylem containing varying amount of secondary structures depending on age.

GROUND TISSUE large, parenchymatous cells resembling those of cortex.

Note: Volatile oil may not be seen in the dried samples though reported to be present in the cells of endodermal layer.

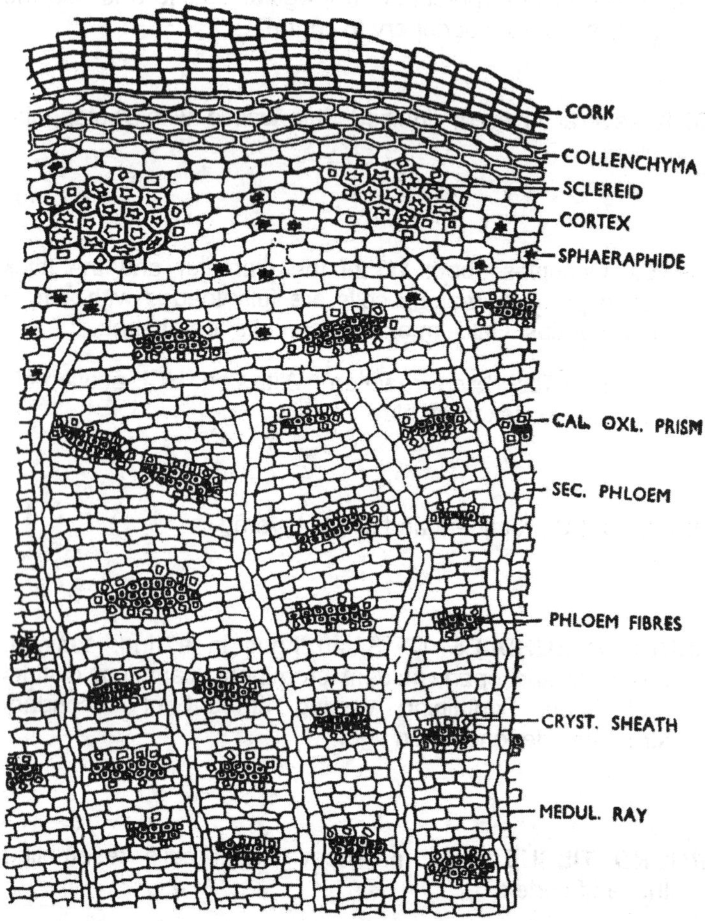

Cascara Bark. T. S. (X 100)

CORTEX CASCARA

(*Rhamnus purshiana* DC.)

T.S. shows a thin periderm, a narrow cortex and a wide secondary phloem.

PERIDERM

Cork 10-15 layers, cells rectangular and arranged regularly in radial rows and have some reddish brown contents.

Phellogen and Phelloderm are not seen clearly.

CORTEX relatively narrow, cells from the outer few layers collenchymatous and the rest parenchymatous. Groups of sclereids which are ovoid to irregular in shape and yellowish in colour are scattered in the parenchyma of the cortex. Parenchymatous cells encircling the groups of sclereids contain prisms of calcium oxalate. Besides, cluster crystals (sphaeraphides) are also found scattered in the cortical parenchyma.

SECONDARY PHLOEM This region comprises of phloem parenchyma, phloem fibres and medullary rays.

Phloem parenchyma forms the bulk of secondary phloem, cells are small and rounded containing a few minute starch grains. Groups of sclereids as in the cortex may also be found, though not common, in the phloem parenchyma.

Phloem fibres occur in numerous groups which are arranged in tangential rows alternating with phloem parenchyma. Each group of fibres is tangentially elongated and is encircled by a layer of parenchymatous sheath whose cells contain calcium oxalate prisms.

MEDULLARY RAYS numerous and traverse radially the phloem parenchyma. The rays are wavy, 2-4 cells in width and extend upto cortex where they become more wider.

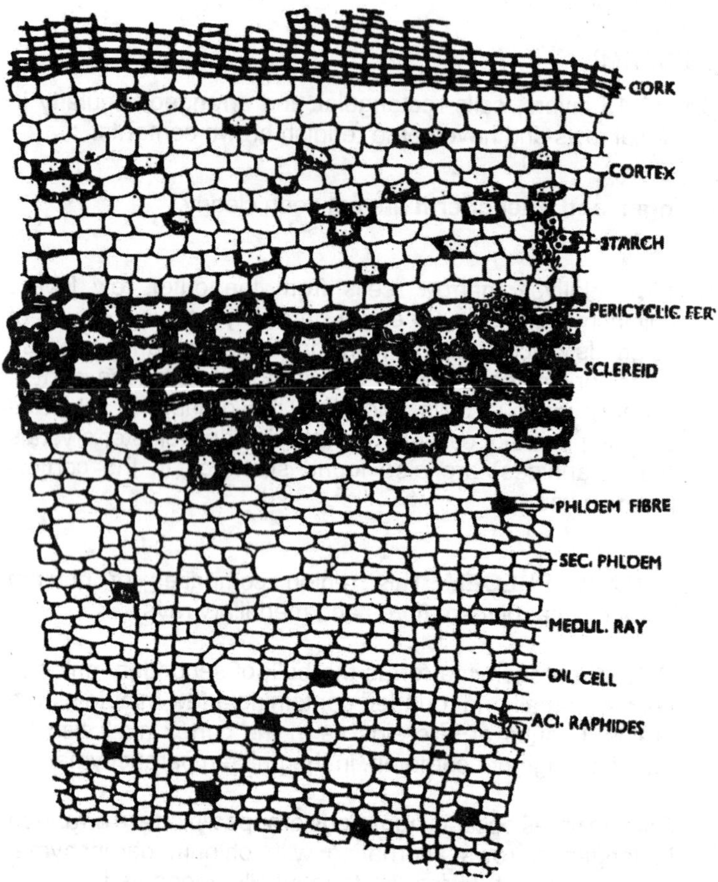

Cassia Bark. T. S. (X 100)

CORTEX CASSIA

(*Cinnamomum cassia* Blume)

T.S. shows broadly a periderm, cortex, a band of sclerenchyma and secondary phloem.

PERIDERM

Cork few layers of which the outer ones are with thin walls and the inner ones are lignified and thick walled.

Phellogen and Phelloderm cannot be distinguished either from each other or from the cork.

CORTEX consists of 10-15 layers of parenchyma in which are scattered sclereids either isolated or in groups. Each sclereid is more or less rectangular and pitted with thickened inner and radial walls. Some of the parenchymatous cells contain minute acicular raphides and abundant starch.

SCLERENCHYMATOUS BAND or STONE CELL LAYER

A continuous well developed belt of sclereids occurs in between the primary cortex and secondary phloem. The sclereids which are lignified and pitted are typical and characteristic of *Cassia* bark. As mentioned above, the inner and radial walls of the sclereids are more thicker than the outer walls giving the appearance of the letter 'U'. On the outerside of the sclerenchymatous band are found a few groups of small pericyclic fibres.

SECONDARY PHLOEM This region comprises of phloem parenchyma, phloem fibres and medullary rays.

Phloem parenchyma consists of thin walled cells containing abundant starch and few minute acicular raphides. Numerous, big isolated oil cells are seen frequently in the phloem parenchyma which is again a characteristic feature of *Cassia* bark.

Phloem fibres occur mostly single and isolated, rarely in groups of 2 to 3, embedded in phloem parenchyma. The fibres are almost circular and lignified with stratification.

MEDULLARY RAYS divide radially several times the phloem parenchyma; 1-3 cells wide and externally extend up to the stone cell layer where they become wider. Ray cells also contain starch and acicular raphides.

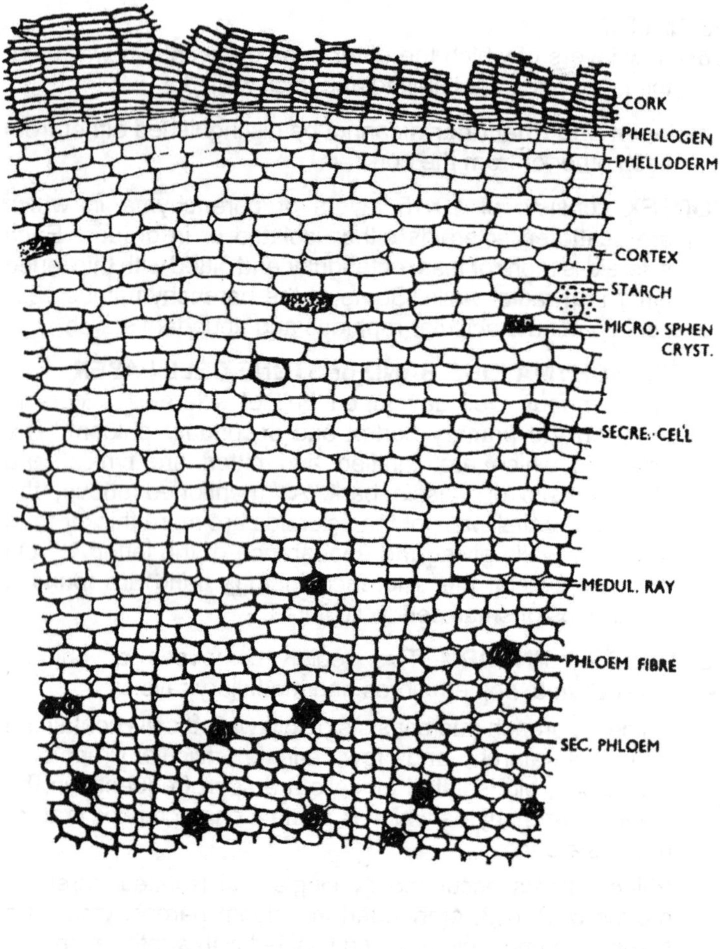

Cinchona Bark. T. S. (X 100)

CORTEX CINCHONA

(*Cinchona sps.*)

T.S. shows a well developed periderm, a wide cortex and a large secondary phloem.

PERIDERM

Cork consists of several layers of radially arranged rows of thin walled cells with dark brown contents. The cork cells are impregnated with suberin.

Phellogen 2 – 3 layers of thin walled rectangular cells without any cell contents.

Phelloderm 6 – 8 layers of thin walled rectangular cells without any cell contents, like cork, they are arranged at times in radial rows.

CORTEX several layers of thin walled and tangentially elongated cells containing yellowish brown matter. Some of the cortical cells are filled with microsphenoidal crystals of calcium oxalate and the rest with minute starch grains. Besides, isolated secretion cells (latex ducts) are also found in the cortical parenchyma.

SECONDARY PHLOEM This region comprises of phloem parenchyma, phloem fibres and medullary rays.

Phloem fibres, characteristic of Cinchona bark occur intermingled with phloem parenchyma and in between medullary rays. Fibres are numerous, mostly isolated, at times in groups of 2 or 3, rounded to oval, in various sizes, yellow in colour, thick walled, strongly lignified with a small lumen and stratifications.

MEDULLARY RAYS traverse radially the phloem parenchyma; 1-3 cells wide, extend upto cortex, cells radially elongated and contain starch grains.

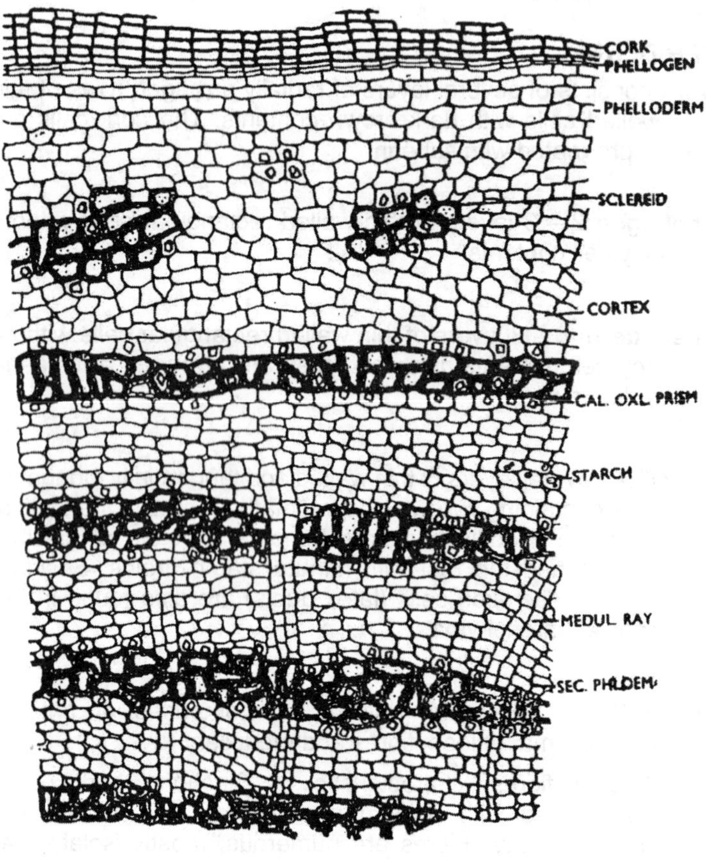

Kurchi Bark. T. S. (X 100)

CORTEX KURCHI

(*Holarrhena antidysenterica* Wall.)

T.S. shows periderm, a wide cortex and secondary phloem.

PERIDERM

Cork 5 to 8 layers, thin walled rectangular cells, some with yellowish matter.

Phellogen 2 layers of colourless rectangular cells.

Phelloderm 6 to 10 layers, thin walled somewhat rectangular cells, at times arranged in radial rows. The parenchymatous cells contain rhomboidal crystals and a few starch grains.

CORTEX wide, interspersed with groups of lignified, pitted, stone cells of large lumen and of various shapes (rectangular to elongated) and sizes. At times, these groups of stone cells form a continuous band. The cortical parenchyma surrounding the stone cells and as well the stone cells themselves contain rhomboidal crystals, a characteristic feature of *Kurchi bark*. Besides, starch grains are found in most of the cortical parenchyma. Occasionally one or two groups of non-lignified pericyclic fibres are seen in the cortex.

SECONDARY PHLOEM This region comprises of mostly phloem parenchyma, medullary rays (not uniformly arranged and appear to run in different directions) and groups of stone cells arranged in tangential rows separated by medullary rays. The stone cells in the secondary phloem region also, are encircled by a sheath of parenchyma containing rhomboidal crystals of calcium oxalate.

MEDULLARY RAYS are one to three seriate, wide towards the outside and consist of thin walled radially elongated parenchymatous cells. Phloem parenchyma and medullary ray cells contain starch grains. Few rhomboidal crystals are seen scattered in the phloem parenchyma. Phloem fibres absent.

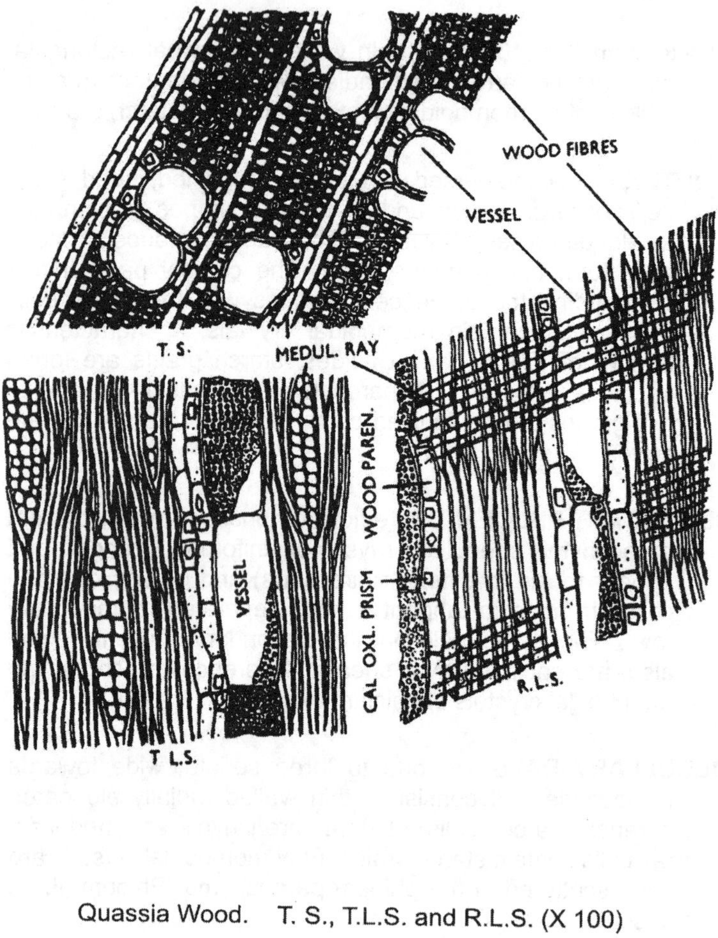

Quassia Wood. T. S., T.L.S. and R.L.S. (X 100)

LIGNUM QUASSIA (*Picrasma excelsa* Benth) also (*Picroena excelsa/Aeschrion excelsa*)

Wood anatomy is studied by taking microscopic sections in three different aspects namely, transverse, tangential longitudinal and radial longitudinal sections.

In a t.s. the following are seen and being wood all the tissues are lignified.

SECONDARY XYLEM consisting of:

(a) **Vessels** big, occurring in large numbers, either single or in groups of few. At times the vessels occupy the entire region between two consecutive medullary rays.

(b) **Wood fibres** form the bulk of the wood, thick walled, pitted and arranged in radial rows and

(c) **Wood parenchyma** small, polygonal with uniformly thickened pitted walls (less thickened than that of fibres). Some cells of wood parenchyma contain prisms of calcium oxalate and few starch grains.

MEDULLARY RAYS prominent, uni-to tetra seriate; ray cells radially elongated, pitted with oblique septa occasionally containing prisms of calcium oxalate and few starch grains.

TANGENTIAL LONGITUDINAL SECTION (TLS) (A longitudinal section taken at the peripheral region of wood)

SECONDARY XYLEM consists of:

(a) **Vessels** wide and elongated showing minute bordered pits and

(b) **Wood fibres** in groups, long and tapering with small oblique bordered pits and

(c) **Wood parenchyma** elongated and have pitted walls. Calcium oxalate prisms are clearly seen in the cells of wood parenchyma in a TLS.

MEDULLARY RAYS are cut transversely and as a result, the height (11-13 cells) and width (1-3 cells) of medullary rays can be made out.

RADIAL LONGITUDINAL SECTION (RLS) (A longitudinal section taken diagonally from the periphery to the centre).

SECONDARY XYLEM same as that of TLS.

MEDULLARY RAYS in groups, crossing the fibres and vessels at right angles. Here the height of the medullary rays can be counted.

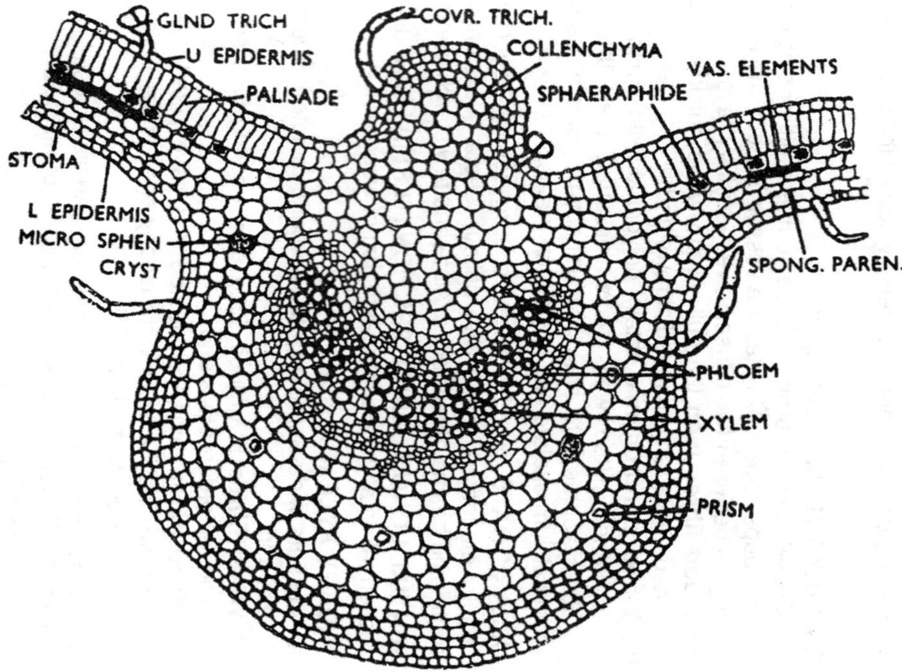

Datura Leaf. T. S. (X 50)

FOLIA DATURA *(Datura sps.)*

T.S. shows a bifacial structure. Following are the important tissues in the lamina and the midrib region:

LAMINA

Upper Epidermis single layered, cells rectangular with cuticularized outer walls. Trichomes, both covering and glandular are seen. Covering trichomes are uniseriate, multicellular, warty and blunt at the apex. Glandular trichomes are made up of a stalk of one cell and a 2 to 4 celled glandular head.

Mesophyll is differentiated into palisade and spongy parenchyma.

Palisade single layered, compact and cells radially elongated.

Spongy Parenchyma many layered, loosely arranged with intercellular spaces, cluster crystals (sphaeraphides), microsphenoidal crystals and vascular strands are found in the upper layers of spongy parenchyma.

Lower Epidermis is identical to upper epidermis. Stomata and numerous trichomes are seen on the lower epidermis.

MIDRIB epidermal layers of lamina are continuous in the midrib region also. Strips of collenchyma appear below the upper and above the lower epidermis. This is followed by cortical parenchyma containing prisms of calcium oxalate and microsphenoidal crystals embedded in the central region of the cortical parenchyma is a bicollateral bundle.

Surface preparation shows Cruciferous stomata and covering and glandular trichomes.

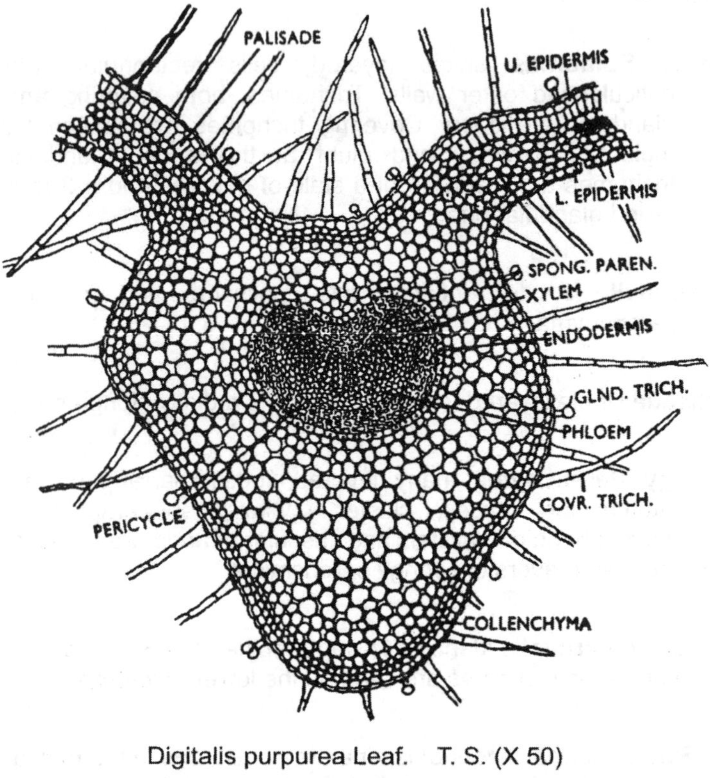

Digitalis purpurea Leaf. T. S. (X 50)

FOLIA DIGITALIS (*Digitalis purpurea* L.)

A T.S. of Folia **D. purpurea** shows dorsiventral nature. Following are the important tissues in the lamina and the midrib region:

LAMINA

Upper Epidermis single layered with more or less rectangular cells having a distinct cuticle. Abundant covering and glandular trichomes emerge from the upper epidermal layer. Covering trichomes are uniseriate, multicellular (3-5-7 celled), mostly straight, warty and with blunt tips. Certain cells of the covering trichomes are collapsed, thus forming a diagnostic feature for the identification. Glandular trichomes are with both unicellular and multicellular (though rare) stalk having unicellular or bicellular terminal gland. Few stomata are also seen on the upper epidermis.

Mesophyll is differentiated into palisade and spongy parenchyma. Calcium oxalate crystals of any type are absent.

Palisade one layered, compact with radially elongated cells.

Spongy Parenchyma 4-6 layered and many distinct obliquely cut veinlets are seen.

Lower Epidermis similar to upper epidermis and has many stomata and more trichomes compared to those of upper epidermis.

MIDRIB The dorsal surface of the midrib is strongly convex and as usual the epidermal layers of lamina continue over the midrib. Below the upper epidermis and above the lower epidermis are seen thin strips of collenchyma. Rest of the midrib is filled with cortical parenchyma. An arc shaped vascular bundle is present more towards the ventral surface (upper epidermis) of the midrib. The vascular bundle is surrounded by a distinct endodermal layer, the cells of which contain abundant starch. Within the endodermis, appears a band of collenchymatous pericycle. Distinct phloem tissue can be seen on the dorsal surface and well developed xylem tissue towards the ventral surface of the midrib.

Surface preparation shows Ranunculaceous type of stomata, less wavy walls of upper epidermal cells and more pronounced wavy walls of lower epidermis and trichomes.

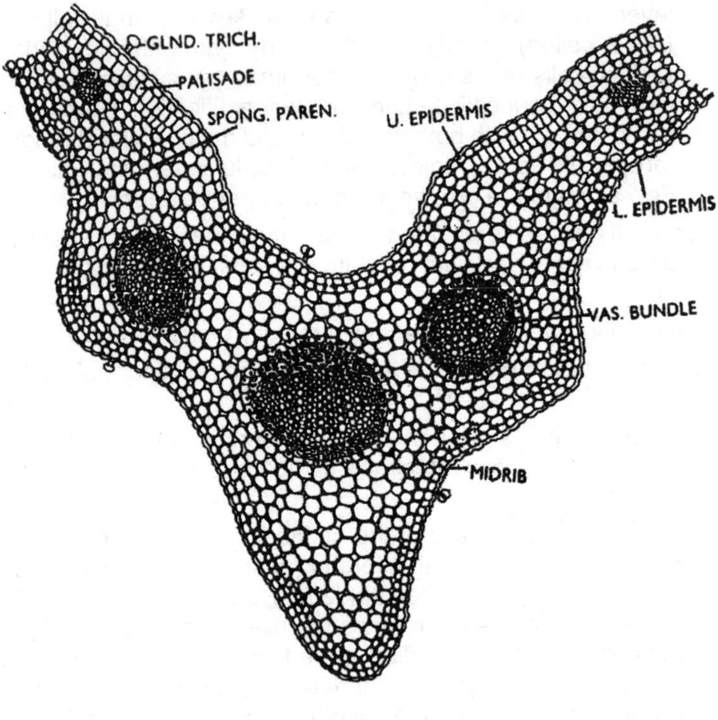

D. lanata Leaf. T. S. (X 50)

FOLIA DIGITALIS (*Digitalis lanata* Ehrh.)

T.S. shows a bifacial structure. Following are the tissues present in the lamina and the midrib region:

LAMINA Because of the prominent secondary veins, the lamina shows frequent projections on the dorsal side.

Upper Epidermis single layered, covered with a thick cuticle, cells have wavy and thick walls; two kinds of trichomes are seen, multicellular, uniseriate covering trichomes (very rare) and glandular trichomes with unicellular stalk and uni or bicellular head (compared to D. *purpurea*, the glandular trichomes are very few). Stomata are also seen occasionally on the upper epidermis.

Mesophyll is differentiated into palisade and spongy parenchyma. Calcium oxalate crystals of any type are absent.

Palisade 2 layered, loosely arranged and does not form a continuous band throughout as it is absent above the vascular bundles of lamina.

Spongy Parenchyma many layered and shows distinct transversely cut vascular bundles as in the midrib.

Lower Epidermis identical to upper epidermis but has numerous stomata.

MIDRIB almost triangular in outline with a pronounced pointed projection on the dorsal side. Epidermal layers of lamina are in continuity with that of midrib but the cells of the latter are smaller in size. The rest of the tissues are identical to those of *D. purpurea*.

Surface preparation shows Ranunculaceous stomata and irregularly beaded anticlinal walls of the epidermal cells which form the diagnostic character in the identification of *D. lanata*.

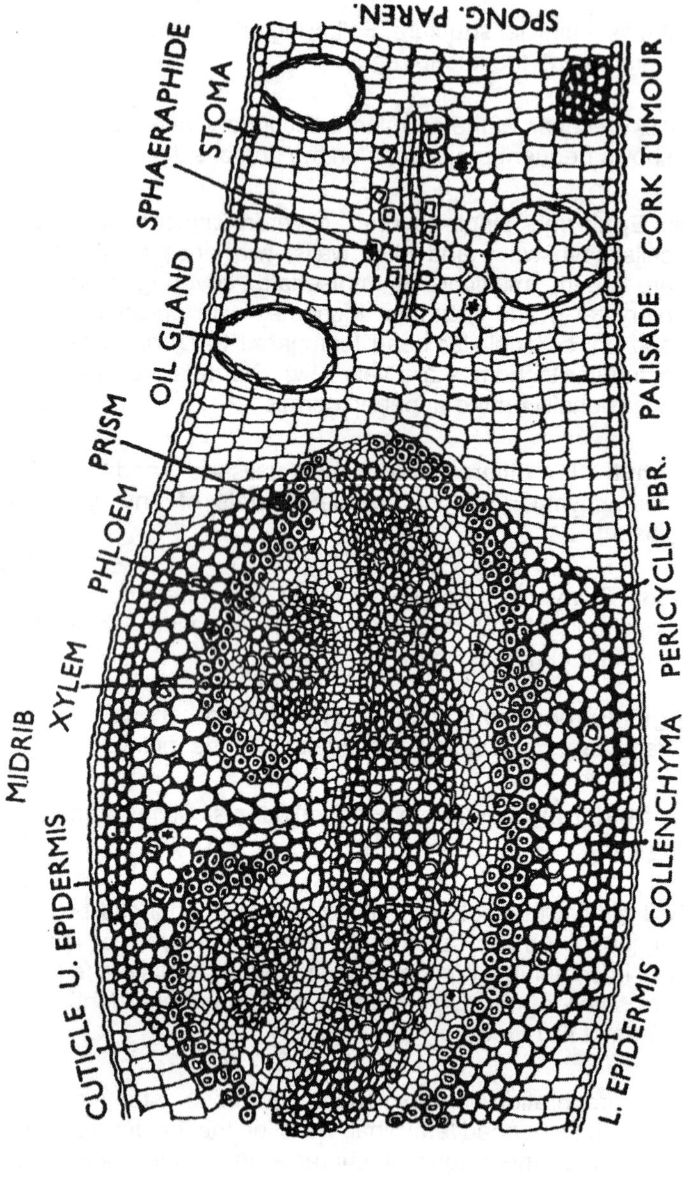

Eucalyptus Leaf. T. S. (X 50)

FOLIA EUCALYPTI (*Eucalyptus globulus* Labill.)

The T.S. shows an isobilateral condition. The tissues represented in the lamina and the midrib region are as follows:

LAMINA

Upper Epidermis single layered with a very thick cuticle, small, rectangular cells and no trichomes of any kind. Sunken stomata are seen frequently.

Mesophyll is differentiated into palisade and spongy and being an isobilateral leaf, palisade is further divided into upper and lower palisade. Schizogenous oil glands, cork tumours (brownish in colour), calcium oxalate prisms, sphaeraphides (cluster crystals) and obliquely cut vascular strands are seen very frequently in the mesophyll.

Upper Palisade 3 – 5 layered, cells are thin walled, compact and not much elongated. Numerous, oval to sub-globular schizogenous oil glands opening towards the upper epidermis are seen in the palisade region.

Spongy Mesophyll 3 – 5 layered, no regualarity in the cell structure but contains calcium oxalate prisms and sphaeraphides. The parenchymatous cells are projected in the same direction as that of palisade.

Lower Palisade resembles upper palisade.

Lower Epidermis identical to upper epidermis.

MIDRIB uniform dorsal and ventral surfaces; epidermal cells of the lamina continue over the midrib. A patch of collenchyma is found below the upper and above the lower epidermis. Major portion of the midrib is occupied by well developed vascular bundles which are surrounded by an incomplete sheath of fibrous pericycle. Xylem from different bundles together forms a bow shaped structure having phloem on either sides. Two more separate groups of xylem elements are seen towards the ventral surface having phloem on either sides and further covered partly by a sheath of a pericycle. Prisms and sphaeraphides are also seen in the midrib region.

Surface preparation shows well defined polygonal epidermal cells with numerous well developed, prominent and sunken stomata of the Ranunculaceous type.

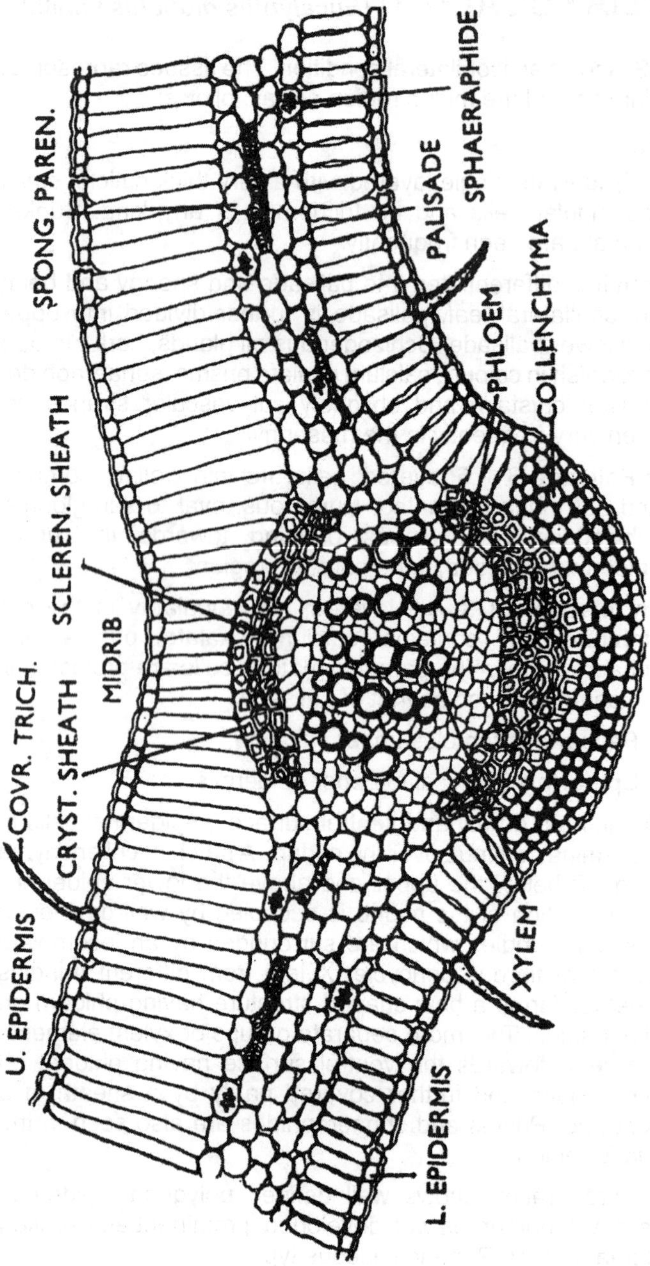

Senna Leaflet. T. S. (X 100)

FOLIA SENNA (*Cassia angustifolia* Vahl.)

T.S. of a leaflet shows an isobilateral condition. The following are the tissues represented in the lamina and the midrib region:

LAMINA

Upper Epidermis single layered with polygonal cells covered on the outerside by a thick warty cuticle. Some epidermal cells contain mucilage. Only covering trichomes emerge from the epidermal layer. Trichomes are non-glandular, short, thick, unicellular, non-lignified, warty and slightly curved at the bulbous base. Stomata are seen at regular intervals.

Mesophyll is differentiated into palisade and spongy parenchyma. Being a unifacial or isobilateral leaf, palisade is further differentiated into upper and lower palisade.

Upper Palisade single layered, compact with elongated narrow, columnar cells and this continues also over the midrib region.

Spongy Parenchyma thin, narrow, loosely arranged between the upper and lower palisade. Vascular strands are seen very frequently. Few sphaeraphides (cluster crystals) are also seen in the parenchyma.

Lower Palisade is restricted, unlike upper palisade, to lamina region only. Cells are smaller than those of upper palisade, loosely arranged and their walls are wavy.

Lower Epidermis is very similar to upper epidermis.

MIDRIB presents a flat ventral surface and convex dorsal surface. The epidermal layers are continuous over the midrib. The cells of the lower epidermis however are small with thick cuticle. The cells of the upper palisade, a tissue which appears below the upper epidermis in the midrib region, are relatively smaller. As mentioned earlier the lower palisade is not represented in the midrib and instead a patch of collenchyma is seen.

Collateral vascular bundle is prominent occupying the central portion of the midrib. Xylem as usual is towards the ventral surface and phloem towards the dorsal surface. The vascular bundle is covered on both the sides (dorsal and ventral) by patches of sclerenchymatous fibres. Characteristic of Folia Senna is that these fibres are ensheathed by a layer of parenchyma, the individual cells of which contain calcium oxalate prisms. Such fibres with crystal sheath can also be seen, if not frequently, in the lamina region.

Surface preparation shows typical characteristic Rubiaceous stomata and polygonal epidermal cells and covering trichomes.

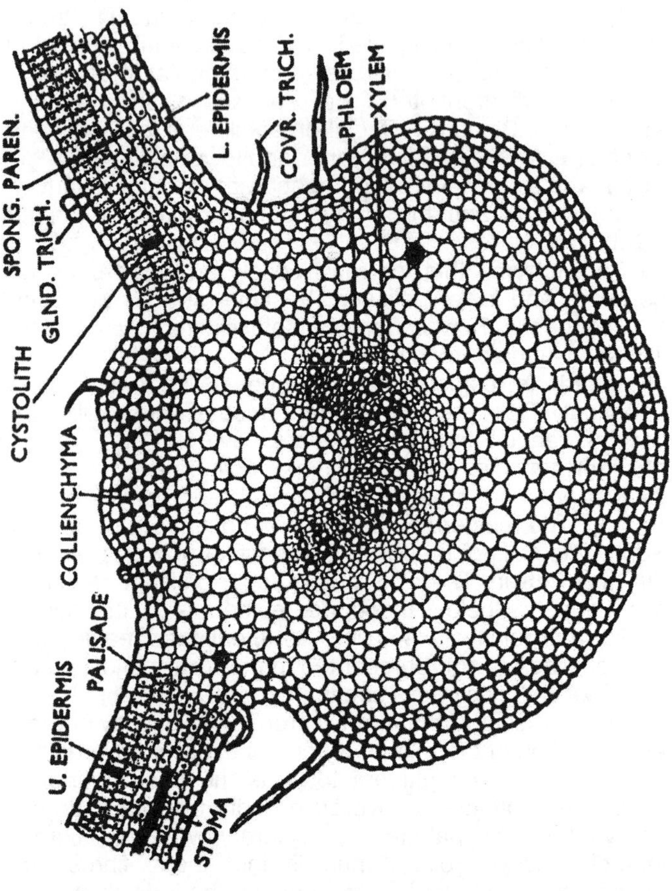

Vasaka Leaf. T. S. (X 50)

FOLIA VASAKA (*Adhatoda vasica* Nees.)

T.S. of Folia Vasaka exhibits a dorsi-ventral nature. Following are the important tissues in the lamina and the midrib region:

LAMINA

Upper epidermis single layered, cells more or less rectangular with outer walls cuticularized. Both covering and glandular trichomes emerge from the upper epidermal cells. Covering trichomes are 2 to 4 celled, bent, thick walled and pointed. Glandular trichomes are sessile with quadricellular heads.

Mesophyll is differentiated, being a dorsiventral leaf, into upper palisade layer and lower spongy parenchyma. A few cystoliths (seen when mounted in water) and vascular strands can be seen in the mesophyll tissue.

Palisade 2 layered, compact and individual cells radially elongated.

Spongy parenchyma 4 to 6 layered, loosely arranged with intercellular spaces.

Lower epidermis resembles the upper epidermis but for the presence of more number of trichomes and stomatal pores.

MIDRIB The upper and lower epidermal layers of lamina are continuous over the midrib. However, relatively more trichomes appear on the epidermal layers of the midrib. A 2 to 4 layered collenchyma can be clearly seen below the upper and above the lower epidermis. The rest of the midrib is occupied by the cortical parenchyma with the vascular bundle embedded in the middle. A few cystoliths can be seen in the cortical parenchyma. Vascular bundle is arc shaped, collateral with xylem towards upper epidermis and phloem towards lower epidermis.

Surface preparation shows epidermal cells with wavy outline, Caryophyllaceous stomata and covering and glandular trichomes.

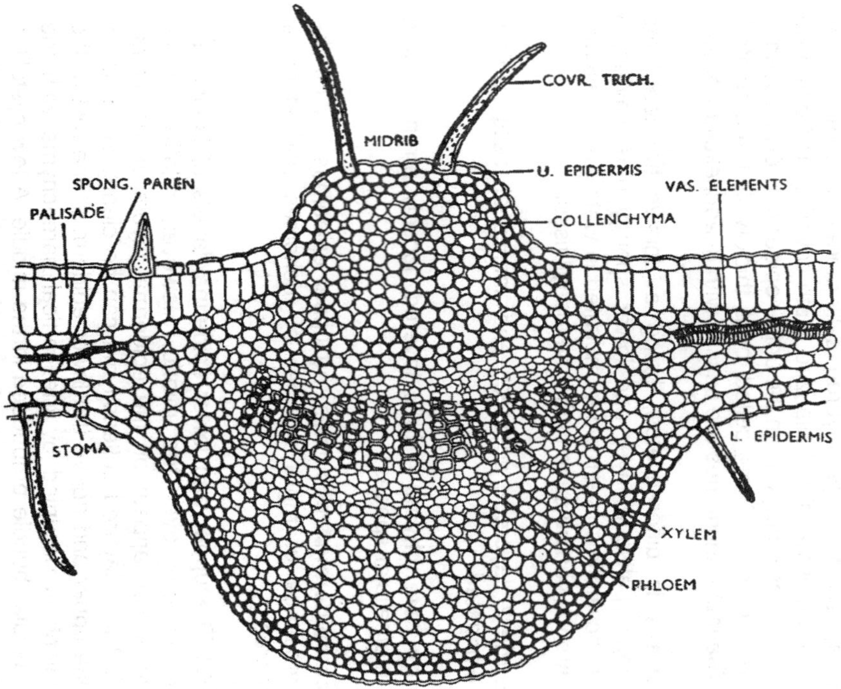

Vinca Leaf. T. S. (X 100)

FOLIA VINCA

(*Vinca rosea* L. = *Catharanthus roseus* (L.) G. Don)

T.S. shows a dorsi-ventral pattern. The following are the tissues represented in the lamina and the midrib region:

LAMINA

Upper epidermis single layered with more or less rectangular cells, the outer walls of which are cuticularised. Only covering trichomes emerge from the epidermal layer. Trichomes are unicellular, long and dagger shaped, warty and with a bulbous base. Sometimes very short trichomes are also seen. A few stomata are seen on the upper epidermis.

Mesophyll being a dorsiventral leaf, mesophyll is differentiated into palisade and spongy parenchyma.

Palisade single layered, cells elongated and compact.

Spongy parenchyma 5 to 8 layered, loosely arranged with intercellur spaces. Calcium oxalate crystals of any kind are totally absent. Vascular strands are seen here at times.

Lower epidermis Resembles upper epidermis but then the number of stomata are more here.

MIDRIB Epidermal layers of lamina are continuous in the midrib region also. Strips of collenchyma appear below the upper epidermis and above the lower epidermis. This is followed by cortical parenchyma. A well developed vascular bundle is seen in the centre of midrib.

Surface preparation shows Cruciferous stomata and covering trichomes.

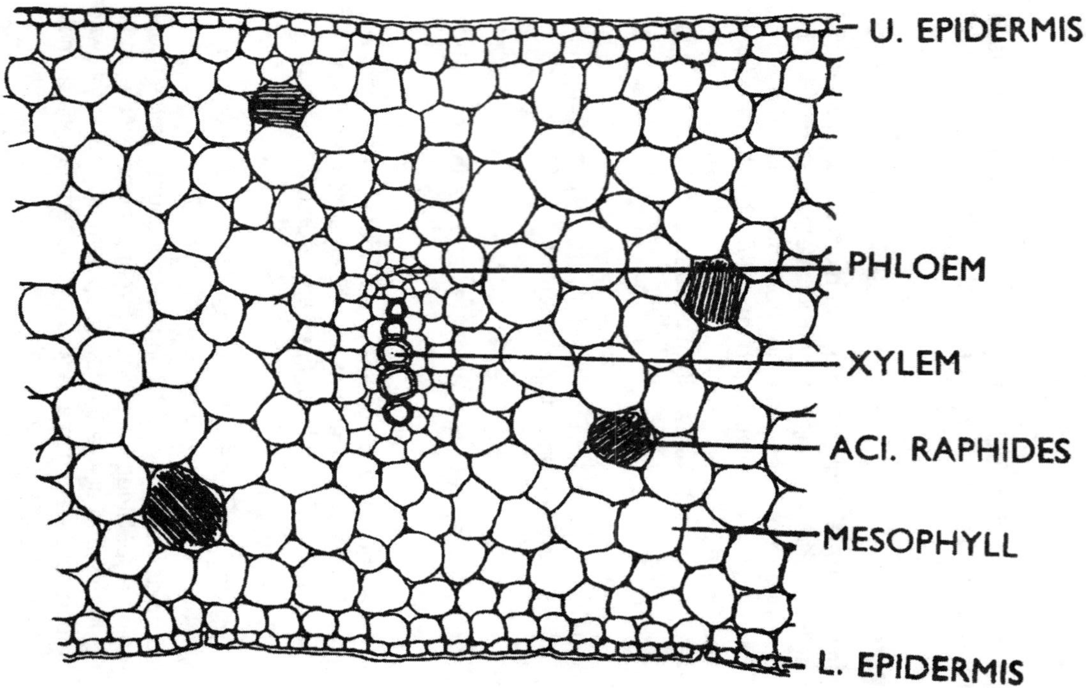

Squill (Scale Leaf). T. S. (X 50)

BULBUS SCILLAE (*Urginea indica Kunth.*)

T.S. of a scale leaf shows an isobilateral nature with the following tissues:

UPPER EPIDERMIS single layered with a moderately thick cuticle, epidermal cells with thin walls, rounded to polygonal at times axially elongated; no trichomes of any knid.

MESOPHYLL forms the bulk and is not differentiated and consists only of thin walled, large, polyherdral, colourless parenchyama with intercellular spaces. Numerous bundles of acicular raphides are seen in the parenchymatous cells of mesophyll, at times still embedded in the mucilagenous sheath. Collateral bundles are seen at regular intervals and has phloem towards upper epidermis and a relatively well developed xylem towards the lower epidermis.

LOWER EPIDERMIS similar to upper epidermis but in addition a few stomata are seen.

Note: 1. The mucilage does not give positive reaction with the usual mucilage stain – Ruthenium Red, instead stains bright red with Corallin – soda.

2. Indian Squill can be distinguished from European Squill on the basis of Iodine water test. When a section of the Indian Squill is mounted in con. Iodine water, reddish purple colour is obtained, whereas European Squill gives pale yellow colour.

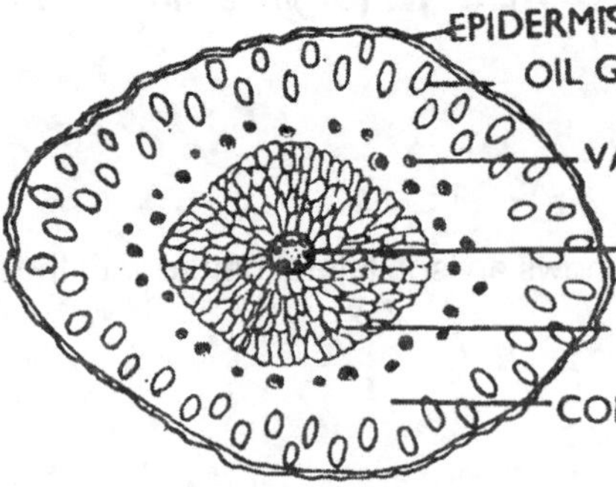

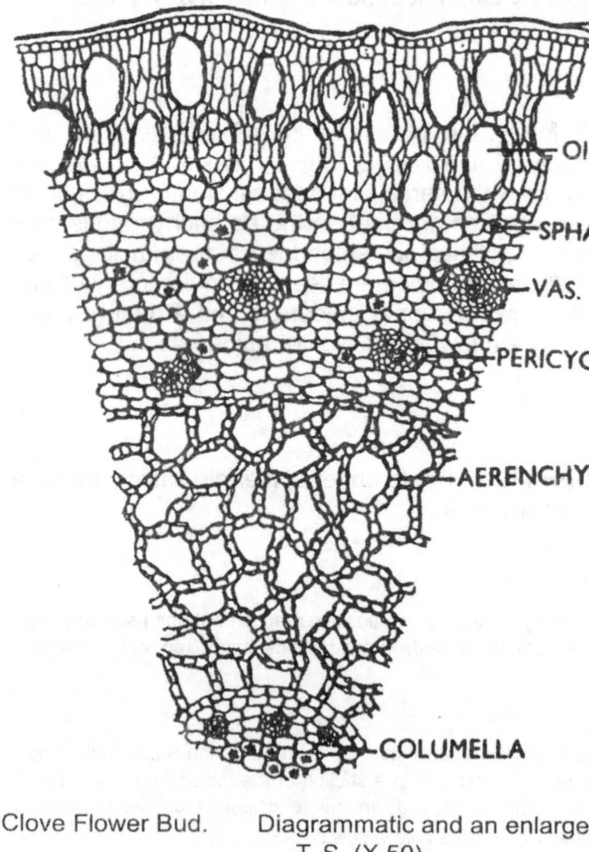

Clove Flower Bud. Diagrammatic and an enlarged portion of T. S. (X 50)

FLORES CARYOPHYLLI

(Syzygium aromaticum* (L) *Merill et. L.M. Perry/ Eugenia caryophyllata Thunb.)

Transverse sections should be taken both through the short upper portion (immediately below the calyx) containing bilocular ovary and as well through the long solid, subcylindrical lower portion (hypanthium) of the bud. Herein a detailed descriptive account of the t.s. through hypanthium only is given.

T.S. through Hypanthium. Following are the important tissues from the periphery to the centre:

Epidermis, Cortex and Columella.

EPIDERMIS single layered small cells with straight walls and has a very thick cuticle. Epidermal layer gets intercepted by Ranunculaceous type of stomata.

CORTEX 3 distinct zones or regions can be made out.

a) The peripheral region containing 2 to 3 layers of big ellipsoidal, schizo-lysigenous oil glands embedded in the radially elongated parenchymatous cells.
b) The middle region containing 1 or 2 rings of bicollateral vascular bundles associated with a few pericyclic fibres, embedded in thick walled parenchyma and
c) the inner region made of loosely arranged aerenchyma.

COLUMELLA forms the central cylinder containing thick walled parenchyma with a ring of bicollateral vascular bundles towards the periphery of the cylinder. Numerous cluster crystals (sphaeraphides) are seen scattered throughout the columella and to a certain extent in the middle cortical zone.

T.S. through the ovary region shows identical structures as that of hypanthium but for the absence of the central columella. This central region here is occupied by a bilocular ovary with several ovules showing an axile placentation.

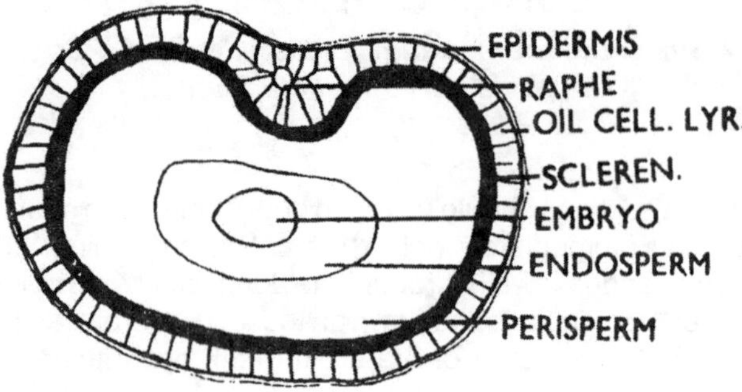

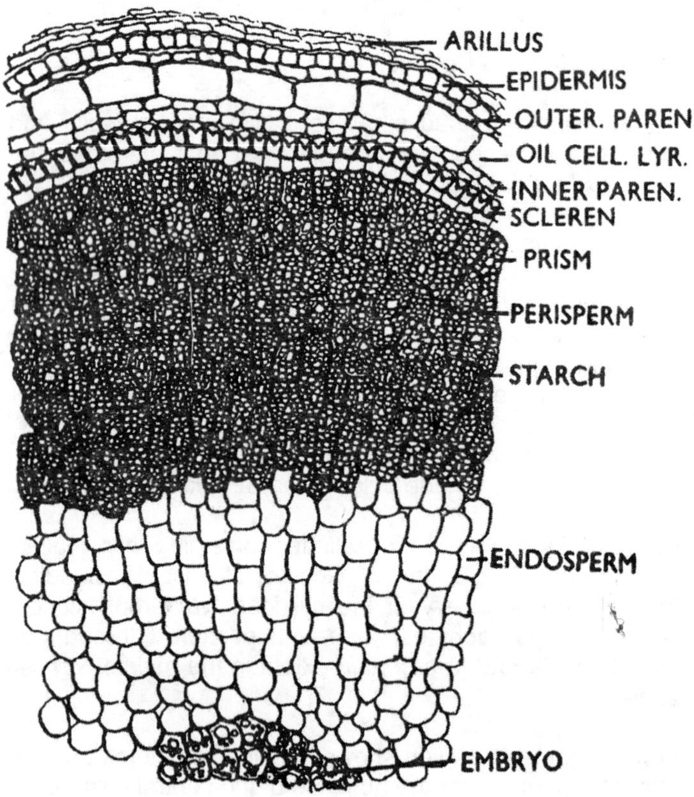

Cardamom Seed. Diagrammatic and an enlarged portion of T. S. (X 100)

FRUCTUS CARDAMOMI

***[Elettaria cardamomum* (White et Maton)]**

T.S. of a seed shows testa, perisperm and endosperm as important tissues.

TESTA The entire testa is covered on the external side by thin colourless, flattened or collapsed parenchyma also called as 'membraneous arillus'. Testa can be broadly divided into outer and inner integuments.

OUTER INTEGUMENT

(a) **Epidermis** single layered, thick walled, narrow and axially elongated cells.

(b) **Outer parenchymatous layer** 1 or 2 layers, tangentially elongated cells.

(c) **Oil cell layer** single layered which however becomes 2 – 3 layered near raphe, large rectangular thin walled parenchymatous cells containing volatile oil.

(d) **Inner parenchymatous layer** several layers of thin walled often obliterated parenchyma.

INNER INTEGUMENT

(a) **Sclerenchymatous layer** dark brown, single layered bowl-shaped cells, radially elongated with anticlinal and inner walls very strongly thickened thus exhibiting a narrow lumen, in which are present nodules of silica.

(b) **Parenchyma** single layered flattened cells.

PERISPERM several layered thin walled parenchymatous cells packed with starch grains and single prisms of calcium oxalate.

ENDOSPERM thin walled colourless parenchymatous cells containing masses of protein.

EMBRYO small cells containing aleurone grains.

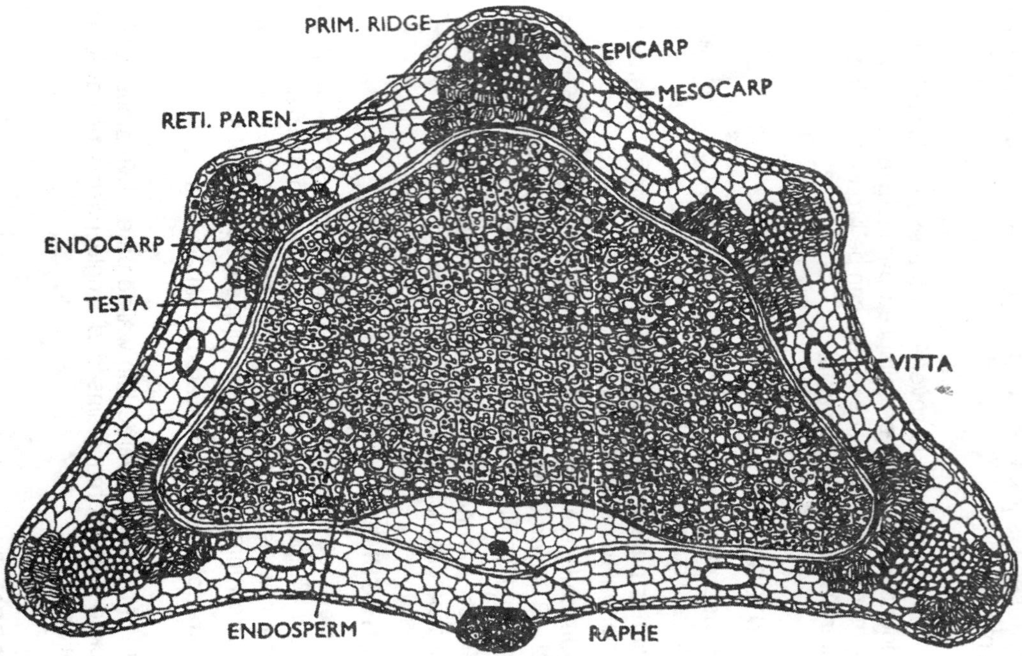

Fennel Fruit. T. S. of Mericarp (X 50)

FRUCTUS FOENICULI *(Foeniculum vulgare* Mill.*)*

Fennel exhibits features of a typical umbelliferous fruit CREMOCARP. When a **schizocarp** (a fruit which splits apart into parts without further dehiscion) is derived from a bicarpellary pistil, it is called a **cremocarp.** In other words, a cremocarp consists of two portions each of which is called a **mericarp** connected by a central stalk called carpophore. A single seed is seen in each mericarp.

T.S. of a mericarp shows two prominent surfaces – the commisural and the dorsal. The commisural surface is flat with two pronounced ridges and carpophore in the middle. The dorsal surface is also ridged (3 ridges). Thus, in all, the mericarp shows 5 primary ridges.

Mericarp can broadly be divided into Pericarp, Testa and the bulky Endosperm.

PERICARP

The **Epicarp** or the **exocarp** of the pericarp surrounding the entire mericarp consists of a layer of polygonal, tangentially elongated cells with smooth cuticle.

Mesocarp the bulk of mesocarp is made of parenchyma. Bicollateral vascular bundles appear in the mesocarp below the primary ridges. Reticulate and lignified parenchyma, a characteristic feature of Fennel appears in the mesocarp surrounding the vascular bundles. Besides, yellowish brown and elliptical vittae (schizogenous oil ducts), 4 on the dorsal surface between the ridges and two on the commisural surface are also important features of mesocarp.

Endocarp Another typical umbelliferous feature is the presence of parquetry arrangement (groups of parallel cells arranged in different directions) of cells of endocarp which however is seen as a single layer between mesocarp and testa.

TESTA single layered and yellowish in colour.

ENDOSPERM thick walled, polygonal colourless parenchyma containing oil globules and aleurone grains. A crescent shaped embryo is seen in the sections passing through the apical region of mesocarp. Raphe, a ridge of vascular strand, appears in the middle of commisural surface just in front of carpophore, as the ovule is anatropous (inverted) here.

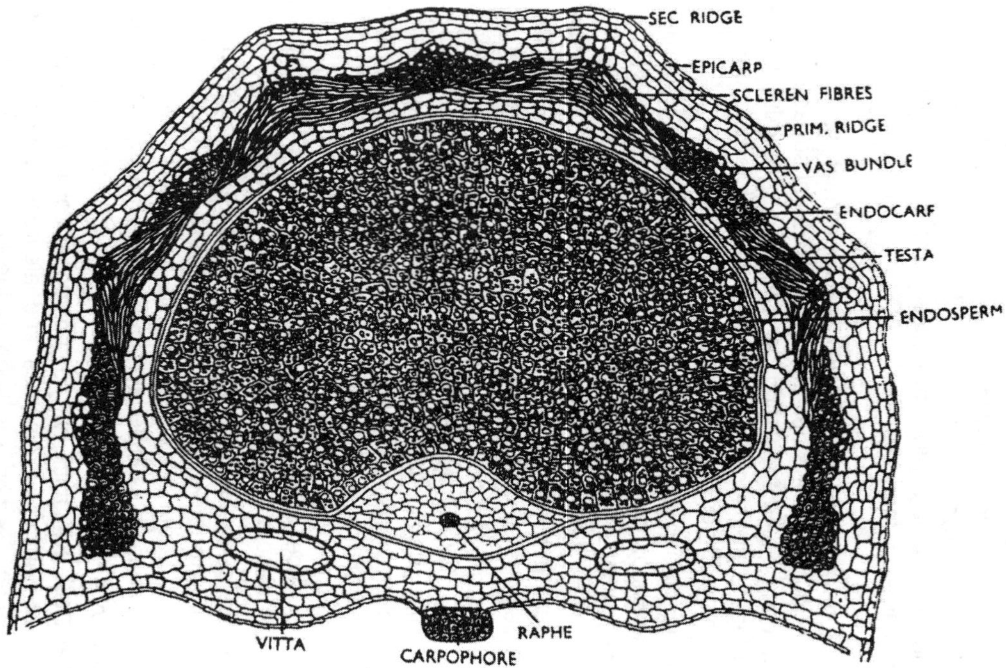

Coriander Fruit. T. S. of Mericarp (X 50)

FRUCTUS CORIANDRI *(Coriandrum sativum L.)*

A t.s. of the mericarp shows two prominent surfaces the commisural and the dorsal. The commisural surface is flat with two vittae and carpophore in the middle. The dorsal surface is ridged but with no vittae. Unlike **Fructus Foeniculi,** here 5 less pronounced primary ridges, and 4 pronounced secondary ridges, each secondary ridge appearing between two primary ridges are seen. Pericarp, testa and a kidney shaped endosperm are the important tissues of a **mericarp.**

PERICARP

Epicarp of the pericarp consists of a single row of small but thick walled cells. (Calcium oxalate crystals are seen when epidermal peelings are mounted.)

Mesocarp can be differentiated into three zones –

(a) Outer loosely arranged tangentially elongated parenchyma.

(b) Middle compact sclerenchyma: outer region of this sclerenchymatous band is represented by longitudinally running fibres (below the primary ridges) whereas the inner region is made of tangentially running fibres corresponding to secondary ridges). Vascular bundles crown the sclerenchymatous region of mesocarp below the primary ridges, and

(c) Inner, irregular, polygonal and lignified parenchyma.

Endocarp or inner pericarp is made of typical parquetry layer.

TESTA single layered and yellowish in colour.

ENDOSPERM thick walled, polygonal, colourless parenchyma containing fixed oil and aleurone grains. An embryo is seen only if t.s. is taken from the apical region of mericarp.

COMPARATIVE ANATOMY OF UMBELLIFEROUS (CREMOCARP) FRUITS

Microscopic Features	Fennel	Coriander	Dill	Indian Dill	Caraway
Mericarp-surface	Dorsal & Commisural	------	Same in all	------	------
Ridges	5 primary of which 3 on the dorsal-and 2 on the commisural surface.	5 less prominent primary and 4 prominent secondary all on dorsal surface.	5 primary ridges of which 3 prominent on the dorsal surface and 2 extending laterally to form wings.	Same as in Dill but wings more prominent.	Same as in Fennel.
Pericarp					
- Epicarp	Single layered with smooth culticle.		Single layered with striated culticle.		
- Mesocarp	Recticulate and lignified parenchyma surrounding the vascular bundle and the rest is made of normal parenchyma.	Outer mesocarp constitutes loose parenchyma, middle mesocarp, a band of sclerenchymatous fibres running longitudinally and tangentially and inner mesocarp made up of lignified parenchyma.	Reticulate and lignified parenchyma as in Fennel.		Parechyma in which are embeded below the ridge and above the sclerenchymatous patch schizogenous canals.
- Vittae in Mesocarp	6 of which 4 are on the dorsal-and 2 on the commisural surface.	Only 2 and are on the commisural surface.	------	As in Fennel	------

Microscopic Features	Fennel	Coriander	Dill	Indian Dill	Caraway
Vascular bundles in Mesocarp	below each ridge, bicollateral.	below primary ridges in association with sclerenchymatous band, poorly represented.	below the ridges, but those of wings are wider than the others.		below the ridges intermingled with pitted sclerenchyma and fibers. Vascular strands consist or inner group of small vessels and fibres and arched outer group of sclerenchyma.
- Endocarp	------	Single layer with parquetry arrangement			Single layer tangentially, elongated cells indicating a week parquetry arrangement.
Seed	Orthospermae	Coelospermae	------	Orthospermae	------
Testa	------	Single layered, yellowish brown occurring below the pericarp			------
Endosperm	-- Thick walled, colourless polygonal parenchymatous cells containing oil globules and aleurone grains ---				
Raphe and Embryo	------	------	------	Present in all ----	-----

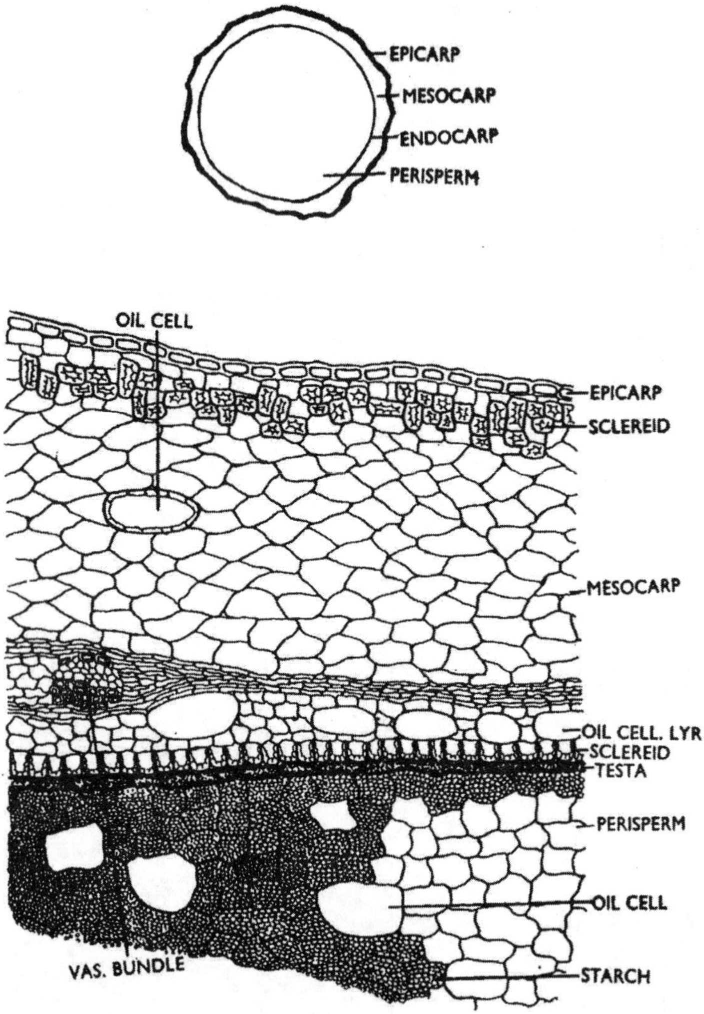

Pepper Fruit. Diagrammatic and an enlarged portion of T. S. (X 150)

FRUCTUS PIPERIS *(Piper nigrum L.)*

T.S. of the fruit shows a well differentiated pericarp, testa and perisperm.

PERICARP consists of an external epicarp, a large parenchymatous mesocarp and single layer of endocarp containing stone cells.

Epicarp epidermal layer of the epicarp consists of tabular cells below which, embedded in the parenchyma are one to two layers of radially elongated lignified stone cells.

Mesocarp is a big band of tangentially elongated parenchymatous cells. Isolated, tangentially elongated oil cells are seen in the outer region of the mesocarp whereas fibrovascular bundles and a regular row of oil cells are seen in the inner region of mesocarp.

Endocarp is made of a row of a beaker shaped stone cells.

TESTA and **PERISPERM** together constitute the seed which lie inside the pericarp. Testa is represented by a single layer of yellow coloured cells. Perisperm forms the bulk of the testa and lies within. Perisperm contains, besides big oil cells, cells containing abundant starch and a few aleurone grains.

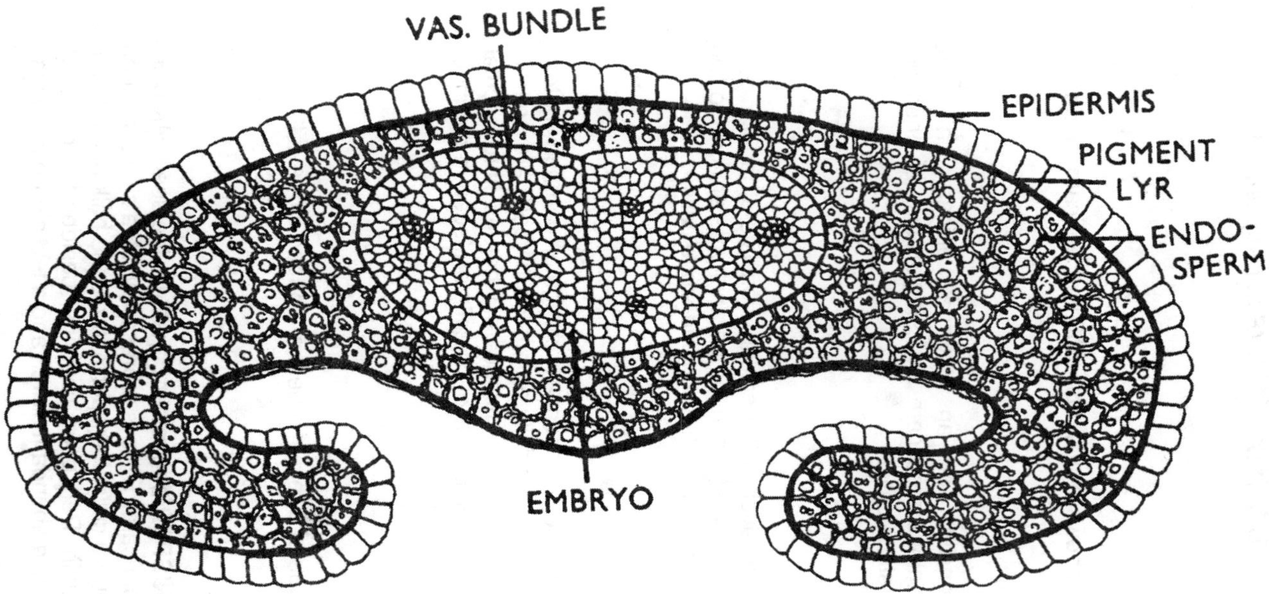

Ispaghula Seed. T. S. (X 50)

SEMEN ISPAGHULA *(Plantago ovata* Forsk.*)*

T.S. of a seed shows two surfaces – a convex and a concave and the following tissues within.

TESTA

Epidermis single layered, colourless, radially elongated, thin walled and shining cells. Because of the presence of abundant mucilage in this layer, the cells swell up when sections are mounted in water. (Mucilage can be stained with Ruthenium Red). The epidermal layer however, does not extend to the hilum on the concave surface.

Pigment layer single layered and yellowish in colour.

ENDOSPERM forms the bulk of the seed, with thick walled, polygonal and pitted parenchymatous cells containing aleurone grains and fixed oil. The cells of outermost layer of endosperm however are palisade like in shape.

EMBRYO is represented in the form of two cotyledons in the centre of the endosperm but more towards the convex surface. 3 or 5 groups of vascular bundles are seen in each cotyledon. The cells of the cotyledons are polyhedral and also contain aleurone grains and fixed oil.

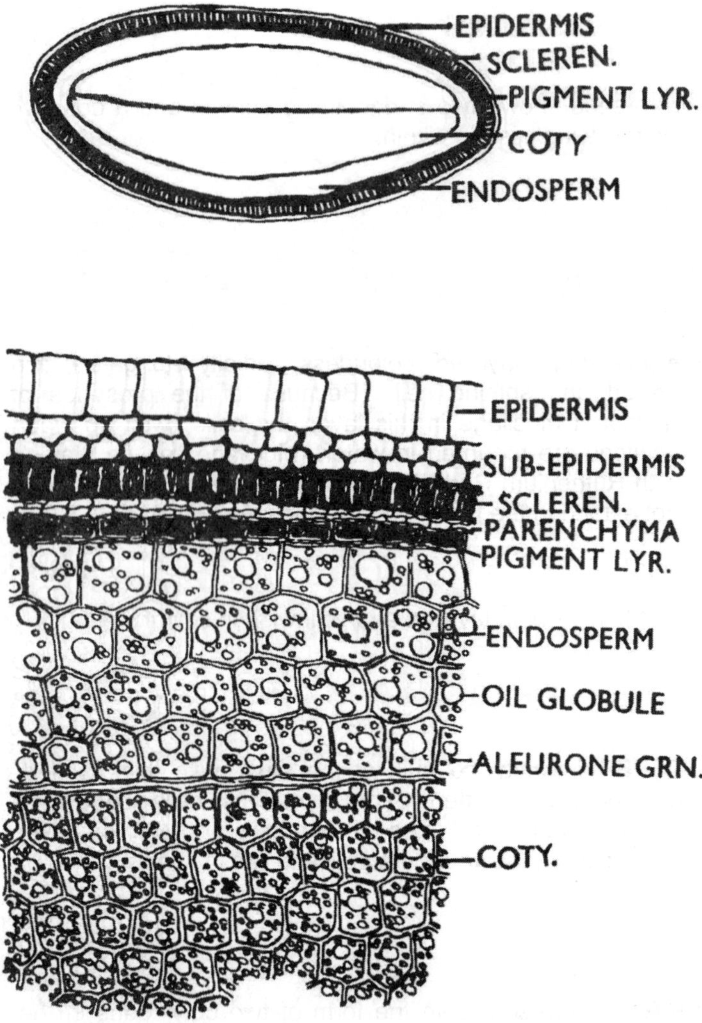

Linseed. Diagrammatic and an enlarged portion of T. S. (X 150)

SEMEN LINI *(Linum usitatissimum* L.*)*

T.S. of seed shows a distinct testa, a narrow endosperm and a pair of bukly cotyledons.

TESTA differentiated into outer – and inner integuments.

OUTER INTEGUMENT consists of –

Epidermis well developed but thin, shining, single layered polygonal and tabular cells with full of mucilage. Ruthenium Red stains the mucilage.

Sub-epidermis 2 layered, yellowish brown, with thick walled parenchyma (collenchyma).

INNER INTEGUMENT comprises of

Sclerenchymatous layer reddish brown, single layered, longitudinally or radially elongated, compactly arranged, lignified stone cells. The cells besides being thick walled are pitted and show a very small lumen.

Parenchymatous layer 1 or 2, with thin, tangentially elongated, collapsed parenchymatous cells.

Pigment layer dark brown or chocolate brown, single layered, thick walled, with pitted rectangular cells.

ENDOSPERM narrow and thin and encircles the cotyledons. The cells of endosperm and cotyledons are parenchymatous, colourless, polyhedral, somewhat thick walled containing aleurone grains and abundant oil globules.

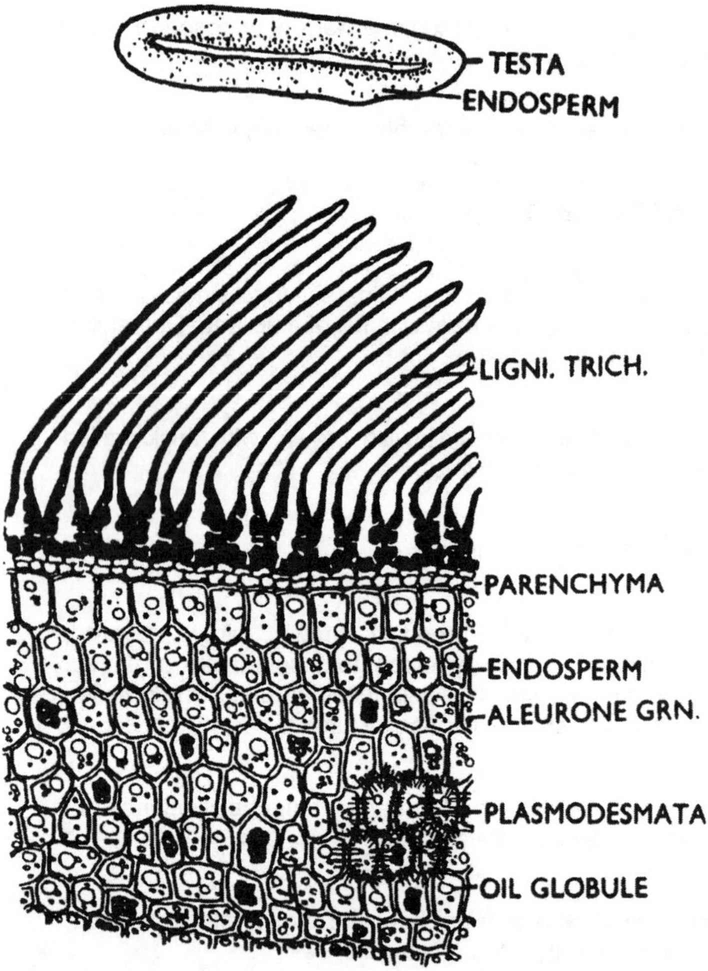

Nux-vomica Seed. Diagrammatic and an enlarged portion of T. S. (X 100)

SEMEN STRYCHNI *(Strychnos nux-vomica* L.)

A hairy testa and a bulky endosperm are seen in t.s. of a seed.

TESTA

Hairy epidermis single layered; each epidermal cell forms a lignified trichome comprising of a pitted bulbous base and a projection which is narrowly elongated and slightly bent beyond the base. The trichomes of all epidermal cells run parallel in one direction giving the testa of the seed a silky appearance.

Collapsed parenchyma 2 layered, collapsed parenchymatous cells with yellowish brown contents.

ENDOSPERM forms the bulk of the seed. Outermost layers of the endosperm below the collapsed parenchyma appear palisade like whereas the inner layers contain cells which are polyhedral, thick walled (cellulose) but un-lignified parenchymatous cells. A characteristic feature of the endosperm of Nux vomica is the presence of well interconnected PLASMODESMATA (fine protoplasmic strands between the different walls of endosperm cells) which can be clearly seen by staining the section with dil Iodine. Besides, the cells of endosperm also contain aleurone grains and oil droplets.

LOCATION OF STRYCHNINE & BRUCINE: Irrigate a t.s. with petroleum ether and add H_2SO_4 plus a drop of ammonium vanadate whereby a violet colour is produced in the central region of the endosperm showing the presence of strychnine.

Brucine, which is present in the peripheral region of the endosperm is detected by staining an irrigated t.s. (as above) with fuming nitric acid whereby a deep orange yellow colour is seen.

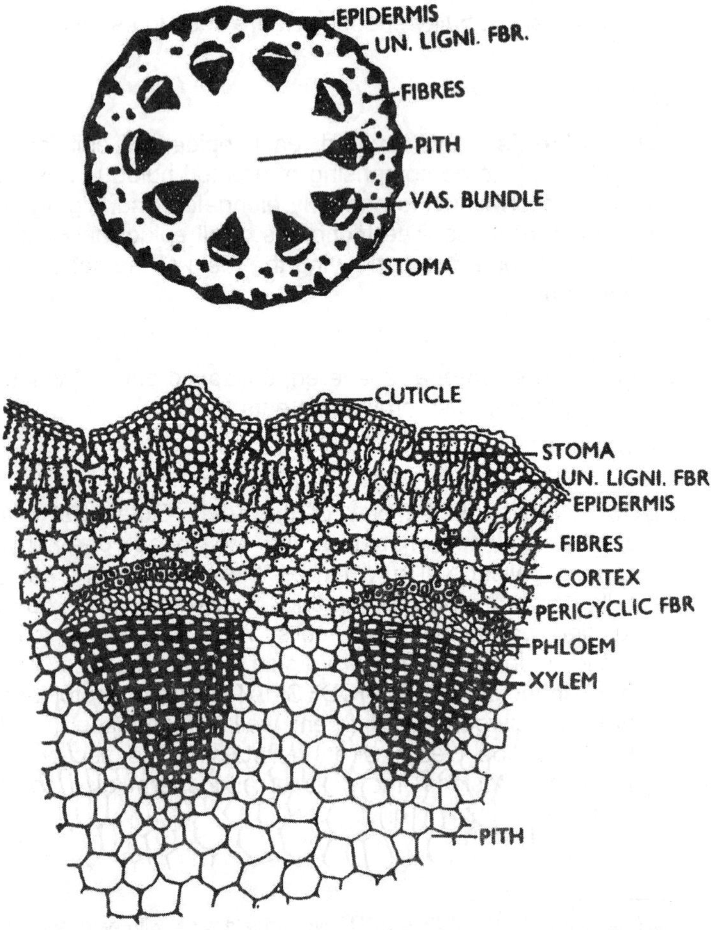

Ephedra Stem. Diagrammatic and an enlarged portion of T. S. through internode (X 100)

HERBA EPHEDRA *(Ephedra sps.)*

A t.s. of the stem (taken through the internode) is more or less circular. The margin is prominently wavy due to the ridges which number from 30 to 40. Following are the important tissues from the periphery to the centre.

EPIDERMIS single row of rectangular cells with a very thick and smooth cuticle. Distinct stomata of sunken type are restricted obviously to furrows.

CORTEX outermost 2-3 layers of cortical parenchyma appearing like loosely arranged palisade cells contain chloroplasts (chlorenchyma). Groups of un-lignified fibres appearing like a bunch of grapes occur below the ridges where no palisade like cells are found. Scattered lignified fibres either isolated or a groups of 2 to 4 occur in the inner layers of oval cortical parenchyma. The latter also shows chloroplasts (chlorenchymatous cells).

VASCULAR BUNDLES around 10, collateral, conjoint, open and arranged in a ring. Phloem is towards the outerside and distinct. Groups of lignified pericyclic fibres crown the phloem on its outer side. Cambium is indistinguishable. Well developed xylem consists of vessels, tracheids, fibrotracheids and parenchyma. Xylem in mature stem shows a well developed continuous band.

PITH is large and is made of thin walled, lignified, big polygonal parenchyma with intercellular spaces. Some cells of the pith contain brownish matter.

BIBLIOGRAPHY

Pharmacopoeia of India : Government of India Publication (1966).

Indian Pharmaceutical Codex : B. Mukerji, C.S.I.R. Publication 1 (1953).

Lehrbuch der Pharmacognosie : E. Stahl, Gustav Fischer Verlag, Stuttgart (1970).

Hagers Handbuch Der Pharmazeutischen Praxis : P. H. List and L. Hoerhammer, Springer Verlag, Berlin – Heidelberg, II (1968), III (1971) and IV (1973).

Text book of Pharmacognosy : T. E. Wallis, J. & A. Churchill Ltd., London 104 Gloucester Place, W. 1 (1967).

Text book of Practical Pharmacognosy : B.E. Hebert and K. W. Ellery; Bailliere Tindall and Cox, London, 7 and 8 Henrietta Street (1948).

Pharmacognosy : G. E. Trease and W. C. Evans; Baillere Tindall, London (1972).

Pharmacognosy of Indian Root and Rhizome Drugs : S. C. Datta and B. Mukerji, Ministry of Health, Government of India, Pharmacognosy Laboratory, Calcutta (1950).

Pharmacognosy of Indian Leaf Drugs : S. C. Datta and B. Mukerji, Ministry of Health, Government of India, Pharmacognosy Laboratory, Calcutta (1952).

A text book of Pharmacognosy : C. S. Shah and J. S. Quadry : Messrs B. S. Shah, Ahmedabad (1971).

State Pharmacopoeia of the Union of Societ Socialist Republics, 9 Edn. Moscow (1961).

Analytical Microscopy : T. E. Wallis, J. & A. Churchill Ltd., London W. 1 (1965).

British Pharmacopoeia : Department of Health and Social Security, Scottish Home and Health Department, Welsh Office, Ministry of Health and Social Services for Northern Ireland (1973).

Pharmacognosy of Ayurvedic Drugs : K. Narayana Iyer and M. Kolammal, Department of Pharmacognosy, University of Kerala, Trivandrum, Series 1 (1-5), (1960); Series 1 (7), (1963); Series 1 (8) 1964.

A Text Book of Pharmacognosy: T. C. Denston, Pitman Medical Publishing Co. Ltd., London (1958).

Indian Journal of Pharmacy (1963, 1964, 1966, 1970 and 1972).

Practical Plant Anatomy : A. S. Foster Affiliated East-West Press P. Ltd., New Delhi (1965).

Comparative Plant Anatomy : S. Carlquist, Hort. Rinehart and Winston Co. (1961).

Plant Anatomy : K. Esau, John Willey & Sons. Inc. (1960).